RATIONING IN HEALTH CARE

The theory and practice of priority setting

Iestyn Williams, Suzanne Robinson and Helen Dickinson

First published in Great Britain in 2012 by

The Policy Press
University of Bristol
Fourth Floor
Beacon House
Queen's Road
Bristol BS8 1QU, UK
t: +44 (0)117 331 4054
f: +44 (0)117 331 4093
tpp-info@bristol.ac.uk
www.policypress.co.uk

North American office:

The Policy Press
c/o The University of Chicago Press
1427 East 60th Street
Chicago, IL 60637, USA
t: +1 773 702 7700
f: +1 773 702 9756
e: sales@press.uchicago.edu
www.press.uchicago.edu

British Library Cataloguing in Publication Data
A catalogue record for this book is available from the British Library.

Library of Congress Cataloging-in-Publication Data
A catalog record for this book has been requested.

ISBN 978 1 84742 774 8 (paperback)
ISBN 978 1 84742 775 5 (hardcover)

Cover design by Robin Hawes
Front cover: photograph kindly supplied by www.istock.com
Printed and bound in Great Britain by TJ International, Padstow

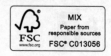

Contents

List of boxes, tables, figures and learning exercises

Boxes

Tables

Figures

Learning exercises

Acknowledgements

We would like to acknowledge the contribution of colleagues from the University of Birmingham and beyond who have helped us develop the ideas presented in the book as well as commenting on draft versions of the manuscript. These include Jo Ellins, Tim Freeman, Sue Jowett, Shirley McIver, Benedict Rumbold and Katie Spence. We would also like to thank the many priority setters and health care managers that we have worked with in our research, consultancy and teaching at the Health Services Management Centre, University of Birmingham.

Foreword

In writing this book, Williams and colleagues revisit a familiar theme in the health policy and management literature: resource scarcity and the pursuit of effective approaches to health care prioritisation. Although the argument as to whether or not rationing is inevitable has been largely settled, there is far less of a consensus over how, and by whom, this should be carried out. Notably, there remains a tension in many health care systems between the rhetoric of governments on the one hand, and the realities of resource allocation at local levels on the other. This text focuses primarily on the local priority setter and is designed to provide both a summary of the major relevant debates and a series of strategies for improving and enhancing practice.

As the authors note, much of the literature on how priority setting should be conducted reflects a dichotomy between advocates of either *information* or *deliberation*. Starting from the premise that both aspects are important to priority setting, the authors assess the contributions to practice that can be found in domains such as health economics, ethics, social policy and the public involvement literature. Coming themselves from a range of disciplinary backgrounds, the authors refrain from advocacy of any single model for priority setting. Instead, the approach adopted here is pragmatic and the book's message is that the choice of priority setting tools and frameworks needs to reflect the aims and contexts of local health services and populations.

The importance of legitimacy and the 'non-decision-making' dimensions of rationing are recurring themes of the book and the authors note that even the most evidence-based and reasonable of priority setting processes is vulnerable to being undermined by external parties. For example, history suggests that local decision-makers are frequently overruled by politicians and/or damaged by media and stakeholder criticism. Furthermore, the gap between priority setting and *actual rationing* – through the closing of services, withdrawal of treatments and so on – often remains pronounced. This is important because, in difficult economic circumstances, elaborate priority setting processes that are neither supported nor implemented are themselves a questionable use of resources.

In this context, *Rationing in Health Care: The Theory and Practice of Priority Setting* makes two important contributions. The first of these is to focus on strategies for increasing the legitimacy and defensibility of local processes. The second is the concern to ensure that priority setting moves from being an often disconnected activity to becoming an effective mechanism for shaping health care organisation and delivery.

Professor Chris Ham
Chief Executive, The Kings Fund, London, UK

ONE

An introduction to priority setting

Key points covered in Chapter One

- Although the rationing 'landscape' may change, many of the main features of rationing controversies are common across settings and over time.
- The terms 'rationing' and 'priority setting' are often used interchangeably. Here they are generally used to refer to different stages of the resource allocation process.
- There are a number of other strategies for dealing with resource scarcity, including: market mechanisms; waiting lists; budget increases; increasing system efficiency; demand and referral management; and implicit rationing.
- Despite the coexistence of these strategies, there is a general trend towards focusing on explicit priority setting.
- This book seeks to assist those charged with carrying out priority setting at local levels of health care.

Introduction

Rationing controversies are a common feature of health care systems throughout the world and have hit the National Health Service (NHS) at regular intervals since its inception. Although the circumstances of these incidents differ, some basic features recur in each case: concerns over limited budgets lead to a decision to restrict access to, or withhold, a treatment, and this decision draws a range of parties – such as the media, government, the courts, charities, industry and the medical profession – into an emotive dispute over health care, its limitations and the perceived failures of those charged with its administration (see Box 1.1 for some recent examples). Although the storm invariably subsides and an uneasy truce between decision-makers and stakeholders is resumed, those hit by the backlash are left in no doubt as to the dangers and pitfalls associated with rationing. Whether it is government, health authorities or health care commissioners, the disincentives for taking responsibility for the allocation of scarce resource are considerable. However, the alternatives – increases in overall investment, long waits for treatment or reliance on the 'bedside' rationing of physicians and hospital administrators – are also increasingly problematic in an era of the expert patient and overstretched public-sector budgets. It could be argued, therefore, that the time has come for explicit priority setting to become a core function of health service planning and delivery. However, the solutions to the problems of rationing remain elusive.

Box 1.1: Rationing controversies in health care

The drug Avastin improves life expectancy for patients with advanced bowel cancer. However, a recent ruling by the National Institute for Health and Clinical Excellence (NICE) adjudged the treatment to be excessively expensive given the benefits it provides. This led to media condemnation (eg Briggs, 2010). Furthermore, Barnsley Primary Care Trust (PCT) was criticised when they refused access to Avastin as a treatment for a brain-tumour sufferer, even though Avastin is not licensed for treatment of this condition (*The Sun*, 2009).

Some years before the Avastin case, a number of PCTs also restricted access to the drug Herceptin on grounds of safety and cost-effectiveness. Interventions from patient groups, industry, government ministers and the courts eventually forced a reversal of the PCTs' position (Kondro and Sibbald, 2005; *The Lancet*, 2005; MacKenzie et al, 2008).

More recently, PCTs have implemented policies designed to limit availability of in vitro fertilisation and/or to impose conditions on patient access (such as smoking cessation) (Hinscliff, 2008). This has led to a high-profile media and interest group backlash (Moore, 2010).

Ham and Pickard (1998) have detailed the case of the family of 'Child B' who were denied a second phase of intensive treatment by the then Cambridge and Huntington Health Authority on the grounds that investing resources in an experimental procedure with little chance of success was not a supportable course of action. Although the High Court ruled that the decision should be reconsidered – on the grounds of the preciousness of the right to life – this was subsequently overturned by the court of appeal.

As a reader you may be thinking, 'That is all very well, but why add another contribution to the already substantial literature on rationing in health care? Is there anything more to be said about the challenges that face priority setters and how these might be overcome?' We would argue that this book provides an important supplement to this literature for a number of reasons. First, the current (and expected future) economic climate has sharpened awareness of the need for effective and explicit priority setting. In the English NHS, for example, recent resource allocation has been carried out within a context of incremental budget uplifts, effectively meaning that decision-makers have been required to choose between new investment opportunities. However, priority setting in a 'cold climate' requires a greater focus on the substitution, withdrawal and decommissioning of services and interventions. This important issue is largely overlooked in the published literature and we seek to address this throughout this text.

Second, a number of recent developments in theory and practice have yet to be brought together in a single text of this kind. For example, this book introduces a range of priority-setting tools and prescriptions – including economic evaluation, multi-criteria decision analysis, accountability for reasonableness and deliberative citizen engagement – and assesses the application of these to practice. Third, we would argue that much of the existing literature fails to fully grasp the underlying drivers of the demand–supply gap in health care, instead focusing exclusively on priority setting as a decision-making function (Øvretveit, 1997). This text seeks to go beyond these debates to look at the non-decision-making elements of priority setting and rationing that, it is argued, are crucial to policy and practice. As such, this text makes a major contribution to existing knowledge though its integration of technical (eg decision analysis) and non-technical (eg politics and leadership) material into a coherent and rounded account of priority-setting theory and practice.

Purpose of this book

Overall, the book brings together theory, practice and evidence from a wide range of disciplines in a way that is intended to be practical and accessible for students and professionals working within contemporary health care settings. It summarises policy and research in a detailed and accessible manner, provides evidence-based recommendations for policy and practice where possible, and maps the major contours of debate where no such evidence presently exists. It specifically seeks to offer support to those working in health care with responsibility for decision-making and priority setting by providing helpful examples and frameworks with which to make sense of the complex challenges they face.

The text is primarily concerned with *meso*-level priority setting: that is, those resource allocating bodies and actors that sit between government (the macro-political context) and individuals (the micro level of patients and professionals). These bodies vary in name and function across health care settings and may include both statutory (eg health authorities) and non-statutory (eg independent non-profit insurers) agencies. In recent years, a number of health care systems have sought to embed priority setting within *commissioning* functions. For example, in England, Primary Care Trusts (PCTs) have emerged as the main NHS payers and therefore the primary resource allocator. PCTs are charged with 'the cycle of assessing the needs of people in an area, designing and then securing appropriate service' (Cabinet Office, 2006, p 4). Arguably, one of the most important aspects of the commissioning cycle is the priority-setting process (see Øvretveit, 1995), and making decisions on resource allocation more explicit to local populations has become particularly important in the context of the present economic climate and future projections of levels of public spending (Appleby, 2008). In these conditions, priority setting can no longer be considered as an add-on to broader commissioning processes, but rather as a set of principles and practices that cut across and underpin all aspects (for more detail on priority setting and contemporary health care commissioning, see Glasby, 2011).

However, just as there is more to commissioning than making resource allocation decisions, priority setting cannot be reduced to the commissioning function. Within the English NHS, for example, priority-setting decisions are also taken by provider organisations through formulary lists, assessment and eligibility regimes, medicines management, and so on, and by other bodies discharging health and social care budgets. In recent times, the National Institute for Health and Clinical Excellence (NICE) has also played an influential role in NHS resource allocation, notably via its economic evaluations of many new treatments and interventions. The commissioning landscape is set to shift once more in the coming years as the 2010 NHS White Paper (Secretary of State for Health, 2010) is implemented.

Overall, the approach adopted in this book is to consider priority setting as a generic activity and therefore to provide insights and information that should be relevant to local decision-makers in a variety of settings. However, many of the examples and illustrations will draw on the specific circumstances surrounding priority setting in the English NHS (see eg Box 1.1). This book is also intended to be useful for a range of audiences – including health care professionals, students and academics. There are some general features that we hope should assist with understanding, including boxes that appear throughout the book with either visual illustrations or examples that ground the conceptual issues discussed within everyday practice. In order to ensure that readers are able to make these links, we have also included learning exercises in each of the chapters as well as summaries of the key points covered. This means that readers should be able to establish the content of each chapter at a glance and therefore select those that are likely to be of most interest or relevance to them. Although a number of key arguments are developed throughout the text, chapters are also structured so as to be self-contained and can therefore be read as discrete discussions of each substantive chapter topic.

Although there are multiple perspectives on (and models of) priority setting, these can be grouped into two broad categories referred to here as 'rationalist' and 'pluralist'. Rationalists advocate rules-based decision-making that is supported by evidence and expertise, whereas pluralists extol the values of participation and consensus in priority setting (Williams, 2011). Much of this book is concerned with the need to incorporate elements of both models if priority setting is to be conducted successfully, and we therefore align this text with those of other authors who have sought to synthesise these sometimes polarised perspectives (eg Holm, 1998; Ham and Robert, 2003).

Structure of the book

In this chapter we set out the key terminology surrounding priority setting and then Chapter Two discusses the *principles* of priority setting. Those involved in the allocation of scarce resources in health care face a number of ethical challenges including the absence of an agreed, single normative principle by which rationing decisions can be judged. This chapter, therefore, summarises the main ethical principles underpinning health care systems and the challenge this multiplicity poses to resource allocators seeking to adopt explicit approaches to priority setting.

One of the key deficiencies of many existing priority-setting processes is the absence of meaningful engagement of the public in the 'tough choices' involved.

There are compelling reasons for this gap, which relate to the difficulty, cost and risks associated with substantive engagement of the public in the complex and highly charged business of health care rationing. However, explicit priority setting requires that this be addressed. Chapter Three, therefore, reviews the literature on deliberative methods of involvement and applies these to priority setting, drawing on theory and research from the UK and elsewhere.

Chapter Four considers the role of economic evaluation in priority setting. It provides a concise, accessible and critical introduction to the theories and methods involved and the application of these to decision-making in practice. Chapter Five then describes approaches to priority setting that attempt to overcome some of the difficulties associated with applying formal economic evaluation techniques. Again, we argue that without an understanding of these approaches and their limits, it is difficult to fully integrate the use of these modes of analysis into the wider governance of priority-setting processes.

The politics of priority setting is the focus of Chapter Six. In order to understand how priority setting takes place, it is necessary to have an appreciation of the political and institutional realities of health care. In traditional 'Westminster'-style political systems such as the UK, health care tends to be subject to considerable reform and regulation from central government. Those charged with the allocation of devolved budgets, therefore, require a working knowledge of the make-up and processes of central government and their responsibilities in relation to national edicts and accountabilities. Furthermore, in order to successfully implement decisions, priority setters require an appreciation of the complex institutional and organisational barriers to decision implementation. Chapter Six, therefore, provides some simple frameworks – drawn from theory and research in the areas of interest groups and networks, the policy process, and organisations and institutions – to aid understanding and practice for those charged with managing scarcity.

Chapter Seven identifies the tasks and skills required for effective leadership within the context of priority setting. Attention is given to considerations of legitimacy, perception and consensus-building in the management of scarce resources. Chapter Eight revisits the specific theme of disinvestment in the light of the issues and frameworks discussed in the previous chapters. The final chapter brings these themes together in a synthesis of lessons and learning for priority setters. Although informed prescriptions for improving priority setting are offered, complexity – in terms of ethics, processes, evidence, organisations, institutions and politics – dictates that any such prescriptions will need to reflect the contingency of priority setting on the local context, and therefore the need for those devising and implementing priority-setting processes to take account of this.

In summary, then, this text is geared primarily towards priority setting at local levels within public health care systems, and draws on specific examples from the English NHS. Less attention is therefore given to the work of either governments or national agencies. Our aim is to provide support to those seeking to overcome the barriers to explicit priority setting and ultimately to help ensure that scarce resources are used in ways that increase the value of health care. The remainder of this chapter provides information on the terminology employed in the text and provides a justification for explicit priority setting as a tool for the rationing of public health care in a context of resource scarcity.

Terminology

Although the terms 'rationing', 'priority setting' and 'managing scarcity' each have distinct connotations, they have all been used to refer to the ways in which health care interventions are restricted in order to control spending or increase efficiency. The term 'rationing' is typically associated with the withholding of resources to the cost of individual patients, whereas 'priority setting' has less starkly negative connotations, referring more to populations than individuals, without directly alluding to punitive resource allocation. The phrase 'managing scarcity' is also used where the resources considered to be finite include both *fixed* (eg organs for transplant) and *circumscribed* (ie the setting of fixed budgets to purchase new treatments) (Klein et al, 1996).

While some authors have retained the distinctions between such terms (eg Klein et al, 1996), others such as Ham and Coulter (2000) argue that the terms 'rationing' and 'priority setting' are, or have effectively become, interchangeable due to the convergence of their connotations. Whichever term is preferred, the implications are similar and involve 'the withholding of potentially beneficial health care through financial or organisational features of the health care system in question' (Norheim, 1999, p 1426) or the 'withholding of beneficial medical care due to economic constraints' (Schwappach and Koeck, 2004, p 1891). Both terms are used in this text, although 'priority setting' is typically applied to an earlier stage in the process of allocating resources. In the words of Klein (2010, p 389):

> Priority setting describes decisions about the allocation of resources
> between the competing claims of different services, different patient
> groups or different elements of care. Rationing, in turn, describes the
> effect of those decisions on individual patients, that is, the extent to
> which patients receive less than the best possible treatment as a result.

Thus, rationing can be understood as the actual impact on patient care of priority-setting decisions. Although the clinical decisions of doctors and patients have resource implications, this text is generally concerned with decisions made at the population level. Population-based resource allocation decisions can be made at the *macro* level (eg by governments) or at the *meso* level (by regional payers, insurance providers etc). Explicit priority setting involves 'identifying systematic rules to decide which patients should secure favoured access to limited health care resources' (Goddard et al, 2006, p 79). In most manifestations, this involves overt determination of either the health care interventions that are made available or the patient groups deemed eligible to receive them. In either approach, the limits of what is to be funded are set at policy levels rather than as part of routine clinical practice.

As already noted, much of the emphasis in the area of prioritisation has been on the allocation of *additional* funding, and there has been relatively little attention given to the substitution of, disinvestment in or withdrawal of services and interventions. Elshaug et al (2007, p 2) define disinvestment as: 'processes of (partially or completely) withdrawing health resources from any existing health care practices, procedures, technologies or pharmaceuticals'.

Although disinvestment can be pursued at any time or in any context, it becomes both more necessary and more urgent in a context of resource deficit and/or reduction. It is possible to hypothesise the following relationship between economic conditions and the tasks of priority setting:

- *Priority setting in a context of limited resource increases:* this requires the development and implementation of criteria and processes for *choosing between* competing service/intervention options.
- *Priority setting in a context of static budgets:* this requires the development and implementation of criteria and processes for the *substitution* of existing practices with new, more effective practices at no overall increase in expenditure.
- *Priority setting in a context of reduced budgets:* this requires development and implementation of criteria and processes for the managed *disinvestment* in existing services/interventions according to agreed criteria.

Following a period of sustained increases in investment in health care, a spending freeze (or even low-level growth) is likely to be experienced as a relative famine for those managing health care resources and the cold climate will become 'arctic' in the event of actual spending cuts (Appleby et al, 2009).

Alternatives to priority setting

Those who argue that rationing is inevitable typically cite the pressure on publicly funded systems created by the growing cost of health care. Indeed, it is difficult to get very far within recent Department of Health publications without coming across the major factors that are seen as instrumental in this: that populations in developed economies are generally ageing and presenting different types of illness and disease in the latter periods of their lives; the unprecedented explosion in costly medical treatments and technological advances; and the rising public expectations of quality and choice in health care provision. The consequences of these increases in demand are exacerbated by the downturns experienced by many economies, leaving publicly funded health services facing an ever-more urgent need to restrict the use of resources. Furthermore, the apparently worsening ecological climate has implications for the *physical* resources that can be deployed in health care provision, and there are ongoing limitations in the supply of life-saving resources such as transplantable human organs (Ubel et al, 1993). Therefore, the notion of scarcity extends to shortages in both natural and financial resources.

In order to survive, public systems have to 'manage the gaps' between demand and supply in an ethically acceptable manner (Øvretveit, 1997). In this text, we support the claim that explicit priority setting is a valid response to the problems arising from resource scarcity in health care. However, it is not the only available response and the assertion that scarcity is inevitable has not gone unchallenged (see eg Deakin, 1994; Evans, 1997; Mays, 2000; Mullen and Spurgeon, 2000). It is, therefore, worth noting the following alternatives to an explicit priority-setting approach.

Rationing by ability to pay

As Goddard et al (2006, p 80) note, the extent to which governments are formally required to overcome the problem of scarcity depends on the level of statutory involvement in health care:

> If a health system were to rely entirely on market mechanisms for delivering health care, the priority setting problem would effectively be delegated to the competitive pressures of supply and demand, without recourse to conscious policy making.

In practice, however, almost no country relies to any great extent on unfettered health care markets. Instead, most health care systems, as they are currently constituted, are the result of central planning and regulation, interest group contestation, and the incremental development of structures and practices. While all countries have a mixture of funding methods in operation, all are dominated by insurance-based practices which involve a third party (either public or private) that collects and allocates resources on behalf of individuals. Table 1.1 outlines the different types of insurance-based systems in operation and the main mechanisms used for controlling spending.

Table 1.1: Approaches to health system funding

Insurance model	Third party element	Mechanisms for controlling spending
Taxation (examples of countries who have this as the dominant method of funding include the UK, Denmark and Finland)	Central or regional governments allocate budgets to regional payers out of general and/or local taxation	Public planning and regulation are the most commonly adopted tools for controlling the introduction of new technologies and services
Social insurance (examples of countries who have this as the dominant method of funding include Germany and France)	Health funds are financed by payroll deductions	The introduction of new technologies is governed by insurance providers, subject to regulation. In this model, insurance providers are not-for-profit organisations
Private insurance (an example of where this method is the dominant approach is the US)	Mixed methods – includes funding direct from payroll as well as direct contributions from individuals and employers	The introduction of new technologies is governed by insurance providers, subject to regulation. In this model, insurance providers tend to be for-profit organisations

A country's choice of funding system is strongly influenced by the underlying norms and values of its society, with some seeing health care as a collective good while others see it as a market commodity that can be bought and sold. While most governments have steered clear of price-based competition, preferring to retain an emphasis on principles of solidarity and universalism, it could be argued that the rise of consumerism in contemporary societies has created an environment that is more conducive to systems marked by privatisation, and support for this claim can be seen in the gradual increase in out-of-pocket payments in health care systems traditionally marked by universality and equity. On the other hand, some US commentators have declared the individual rights-based culture of American health care to be unsustainable and have called for a renewal of collective values of fairness and universality (Tauber, 2002). Even in countries such as the US, which have stronger market principles (ie private insurance markets dominate), funding mechanisms that allow for redistribution of funds to those who are unable to pay are in operation via Medicare and Medicaid, and therefore the government must still make arrangements for scarce public resources to be allocated (Robinson, 2011).

Rationing by delay

Health care systems with universal coverage have, in the past, relied heavily on waiting lists to constrain the outflow of scarce resources (Mullen and Spurgeon, 2000). Typically, such an approach assumes the greater ethical claims of the emergency case over elective treatment. However, lengthy waits can threaten overall efficiency as health care conditions worsen and also threaten to erode satisfaction with, and support for, the broader health care system (Klein et al, 1996). Lengthy waiting times have, thus, become an increasingly unfavoured political response to scarcity in health care. The UK's Labour government of 1997–2010 made reducing waiting times a key priority in the early years of its administration and made significant impacts on the reduction of waiting times for elective procedures. This early focus of improvement in the NHS was widely welcomed as it appeared to address an area of considerable public dissatisfaction.

Increasing the overall health care spend

Of course, governments also have the option of increasing the overall level of spend on health care. For example, between 2001 and 2009, the UK NHS received substantial, real-terms increases in its funding. However, this investment did not remove the need for priority setting in resource allocation. As already noted, much of the funding in this early period went into the reduction of waiting times for elective surgery, which arguably made the need for *explicit* priority setting more compelling. It is particularly difficult to make a case for increased NHS funding in a time of economic downturn, especially as health must compete with other valid claims on the public purse. It may be that the societal importance attached to health affords it the status of a 'special good' (Mooney, 1998), which warrants a higher proportion of government expenditure. However, even those countries with the highest average spend on health care struggle with the need to ration, so it appears unrealistic to expect anything but the most substantial funding increases to have a telling impact on scarcity.

Increasing efficiency in the current system

Another option for decision-makers is to concentrate their energies on reducing delivery costs and eliminating system inefficiencies. This might include: reforming contracting and delivery systems; increasing automation and the technological infrastructure; strengthening management; adopting evidence-based practice and so on (Light, 1997; Øvretveit, 1997). However, there has to be some scepticism over the extent to which these approaches will bear sufficient fruit to close the demand–supply gap in health care as systems such as the NHS have already been subject to multiple interventions of this kind without any dramatic efficiency gains (Donaldson et al, 2010).

Focusing on the determinants of health

Acute care has traditionally absorbed the vast majority of health care resources and this has led governments to introduce reforms aimed at strengthening both the primary care sector and preventive public health. There is some support for the argument that prevention and early intervention can bring about an overall reduction in health care spending (Wanless, 2004). However, there are a number of factors that appear to inhibit this shift from a 'sickness' to 'health' emphasis in the organisation and delivery of care. Perhaps the most significant of these is the strength of interest groups with a stake in retaining the current structures, including the acute sector itself, as well as industries that profit from the proliferation of curative treatments (Jones, 2008; Shapiro, 2010). Furthermore, there is evidence to demonstrate public support for continued investment in acute care despite the potential health gains of redirecting resources towards addressing the determinants of health (eg Yeo et al, 1999), although this is an empirical base that requires much development. While it is widely accepted that health profiles have structural and social determinants, how this should actually translate into coordinated action between health organisations and other statutory and non-statutory bodies is less well understood (Marmot Commission, 2010; Osborne and Kinder, 2011). Achieving substantive change to how health care systems are organised has therefore proved difficult and no system has been entirely successful in reaping the economic benefits projected.

Rationing implicitly

Decisions to withhold treatment or limit access to expensive medicines can be made in an *implicit* or *explicit* fashion. Traditionally within health care, such decisions have been kept 'shielded from public perception' (Syrett, 2003, p 718) in such a way as to render the reasoning 'unclear to anyone except ... the person making the decisions' (Locock, 2000, p 93). Underpinning this 'bedside' rationing is the reliance on the perceived authority of those professionals working at the interface with patients to make decisions. Although funding arrangements have imposed budget ceilings on NHS organisations and professionals working within them, sufficient flexibility has been afforded to enable the concealment of resource rationing decisions behind rhetoric of clinical reasoning and judgement. However, this reliance on implicit approaches has come under increasing attack and doubt has been cast over the appropriateness of individual clinicians and administrators carrying out the resource allocator role. For example, studies have found general practitioners (GPs) to be unclear as to the principles and criteria they employ when determining access to health care resources (Berney et al, 2005). The danger, therefore, is that implicit rationing will proceed according to the discriminatory cultures prevalent within institutions and broader social contexts, operating on grounds such as age, social class and gender (Coast and Donovan, 1996). Implicit rationing, it is reasoned, leaves decisions of life and death subject to the variability and bias of the practising clinician or manager in question, perpetuating the exclusion of marginalised social groups.

Furthermore, commentators have noted that by covertly limiting potential treatment options, health care organisations deny patients recourse to extra services paid for out of their own pocket from the private sector (Mullen and Spurgeon, 2000). These patrician practices, it is argued, also contribute to the erosion of trust in doctors and undermine patient involvement in their own care (Jones, 2004). Thus, implicit rationing is seen as contributing to ill-informed, arbitrary and inequitable resource allocation and as leading to increased distrust between patient and professional. As well as being undesirable, implicit rationing is also seen as being increasingly less feasible in an era of the expert patient (Coulter, 1999) and the replacement of block contracts with activity-based reimbursement of health care providers. Recent proposals to replace PCTs as the primary commissioners of health care in England will see clinicians in England becoming more explicitly responsible for the rationing of health services. Therefore, despite persistent concerns at the extent to which rationing can ever become fully explicit, there is an undeniable international shift towards the development of formal criteria and processes for setting priorities and making resource allocation decisions.

Each of these alternatives to explicit priority setting is problematic in either principle or practice and, when applied, none has been decisive in reducing the gap between demand and supply. Therefore, despite the reservations expressed by some analysts, explicit priority setting is arguably at least as acceptable as these alternatives and therefore a valid option for consideration. Assuming that this proposition is accepted, the question becomes one of how to carry this out in a fair and acceptable manner. This is not to say that these other approaches to managing scarcity will cease to exist and indeed the full range of demand and referral management strategies may well be called upon when resource scarcity

Table 1.2: Involvement in priority setting in public systems

Government	National (and in some cases regional) governments typically set overall budget levels for health. They can also decide on the overall 'basket' of available services or else commission national organisations to do this on their behalf.
Regional and local payers/planners	The role of these bodies depends on the extent of system decentralisation and devolution. However, local decision-makers often play an important role in allocating resources for a local population, either through commissioning or service planning.
Provider organisations and clinicians	In deciding what treatments and services to make available (albeit within the constraints laid down by government), providers engage in resource allocation. This may be carried out as explicit priority setting or implicit rationing.
Patients	Although patients may be involved in any of the above decision-making functions, more typically they may have some input into the resources they personally receive. Through 'individual budgets', patients can be granted a more explicit role in the rationing of their own care.

becomes especially pronounced. In practice, most health systems are a complex weave of explicit and implicit approaches to the management of scarce resources that develop over time and in relation to a wide range of intrinsic and extrinsic forces.

Learning exercise 1.1: Identifying approaches to priority setting

Think about the health system that you are most familiar with and try to identify the different bodies/agencies/individuals that are involved in priority setting at the range of levels set out in Table 1.2. Now try and think of the different types of priority-setting processes and activities that are in operation at these different levels. Are they implicit or explicit approaches? What alternatives to explicit priority-setting processes are in place in this health care system?

Chapter summary

Although the rationing 'landscape' may change, many of the main features of rationing controversies are common across settings and over time. Although terms such as rationing and priority setting are often used interchangeably, here they are generally used to refer to different stages of the resource allocation process. There are a number of strategies for dealing with resource scarcity. However, there is a trend within health care systems towards adoption of explicit approaches to resource allocation. In this chapter, we have detailed the primary focus and aims of this text, which are to summarise and develop the literature on local-level priority setting with examples drawn from the English NHS. In particular, this book is intended to assist those charged with carrying out priority setting and rationing at local levels of health care.

TWO

The ethics of priority setting

Key points covered in Chapter Two

- In public health care systems, priority setting should reflect the broader social values and ethical principles of society.
- There are a range of ethical standpoints that can inform priority setting. These include: egalitarianism, individualism, utilitarianism and communitarianism.
- Other ethical considerations and principles include: desert, rule of rescue, disease severity and fair innings. Each of these has strengths and weaknesses when applied in practice.
- As establishing commonly agreed principles is difficult, more recently priority setting has been concerned with establishing fair decision-making processes. Having a process of priority setting that is seen as fair is also thought to increase trust in health care systems.
- The leading process-based approach for decision-making to have emerged is the accountability for reasonableness (A4R) framework.
- Employing a process model such as A4R does not replace the need for engagement at the level of ethical principles and still requires difficult deliberations between parties who disagree over how resources should be allocated.

Introduction

The need to divide public resources between competing claims for investment raises a number of ethical questions for the decision-maker. Defined simply, ethics are 'principles and values which guide or are realised in how we treat other people, in what we say and do and in the decisions and choices which we make' (Øvretveit, 1997, p 129). As public policy decisions are justified in relation to the public good, they are necessarily based on some notion of social value, and this ethical dimension of rationing cannot be side-stepped entirely through appeals to best evidence, economic efficiency or fair process. For this reason, it is important that priority setters in health care have an understanding of the range of ethical principles that influence, or should influence, decisions. However, in a health care context, it has been claimed that 'many managers are unable to understand the basic intellectual concepts that have underpinned ethical debate for thousands of years ... [and are] ethically adrift in a sea of pragmatism' (Wall, 1998, p 9).

Although this statement is extreme and open to dispute, it is clear that the ethical underpinnings of policy decisions are complex and frequently remain unarticulated. This chapter seeks to explore both why this might be the case and how this lack of clarity might be addressed. It provides a description of some of the main principles underpinning health care and draws out the tensions between such principles. Attempts to resolve the problems of a lack of ethical consensus are then discussed, including the replacement of ethical principles with decision-making processes.

The purposes of health care

Although priority setting has often been presented as a discrete area of activity, it in fact goes to the heart of why health care systems exist, and which social values they are expected to embody, as priority setting is only successful when it reflects the civic ideals and norms of the broader society. However, we live in times of increased diversity and heterogeneity, to the extent that any 'one-size-fits-all' model of public-sector organisation is unlikely to meet the needs and wishes of all sections and groups. As a result, providing care for populations has never been more ethically fraught. For example, one might reasonably postulate that the primary aim of health services should be to increase health, and therefore that this should be the main criteria determining resource allocation (Williams, 1998; Maynard, 2001). However, we might also assert the importance of improving health profiles amongst groups suffering higher than average levels of morbidity and mortality, at the expense of some gain in overall health. Additionally, we may think it important to ensure that health services are equipped to save lives where these are endangered, and to respond with greater urgency where need or suffering is greatest. As with concerns for equity and equality, each of these imperatives would compromise the extent to which priority setting focuses on increasing overall population health. To underline how far priority setting can stray from the principle of health maximisation, a recent survey of stakeholders and experts identified 10 dimensions of successful priority setting and these did not include reference to improved clinical outcomes (Sibbald et al, 2009). In short, 'the purpose of a public healthcare system is unclear' (Holm, 1998, p 1001) and this leaves the rules of conduct for priority setting similarly uncertain.

Unsurprisingly, then, it is not always easy to articulate the principles currently guiding resource allocation decisions, much less assign relative weights to these when they compete for prominence in difficult policy decisions. Initiatives such as the National Health Service (NHS) Constitution (Department of Health, 2010b) and the work of the National Institute for Health and Clinical Excellence (NICE) on social values (Rawlins and Culver, 2004; NICE, 2008) are an attempt to introduce clarity over ethical principles. However, further engagement with aims and principles is required of decision-makers who are charged with reflecting the values of their local populations and translating these into meaningful tools for shaping prioritisation. The next sections of this chapter outline some of the key concepts and perspectives relating to the ethics of resource allocation in health care.

Distributive justice

Although definitions of the term 'distributive justice' vary across different disciplines, its basic tenets hold that the allocation of public resources should be informed by the principles of social justice, however these are understood. This argument dates back at least as far as the writings of Aristotle and his claim that 'If the people involved are not equal, they will not receive equal shares' (Morgan, 2005, p 298). Such an assertion justifies allocation of extra resources to certain groups in the service of moral imperatives that are understood and accepted by all. An obvious example is the health inequalities agenda, which seeks to redress the health profile disparities between social groups on the grounds that these are morally unacceptable in a civilised society (Gwatkin, 2000). The ethicist Norman Daniels has argued that the underlying principle of resource allocation should be the enablement of opportunity and participation for all (Daniels and Sabin, 2008). Therefore, the notion of distributive justice is usually accompanied by an appeal to equity and/or equality between people and populations and involves invocation of the 'common good' as the principal objective of public resource allocation.

However, not all ethical injunctions are concerned with distributive justice. In the medical ethics literature, three other principles are added to prescriptions for ethical health care practice (Beauchamp and Childress, 1989). The principle of *autonomy* emphasises the need to respect individual rights and choices, whereas *beneficence* (doing good) and *non-maleficence* (not doing harm) refer to the need for those delivering services to strive to improve and protect the well-being of those in their care. Furthermore, although principles of justice relate directly to the moral challenge of allocating scarce resources, they can also be invoked as grounds for the protection of individual rights and freedoms (Gillon, 1994). Therefore, the call for a fair distribution of benefits across populations can be pitted against powerful moral principles that are focused on the needs and preferences of individual service users. This tension is often played out in the day-to-day realities of health care and can be most clearly seen in the fissures that occasionally open up between clinicians who believe patient care to be their overriding concern and budget-holders who must decide between the competing claims of patient groups and populations (Sabin, 1998; Tauber, 2002). In an era of clinician-led commissioning (and therefore priority setting), this tension between the general and the particular requires those involved to 'oscillate our gaze' between each imperative (Heath, 1999, p 652).

Egalitarianism

Where health care systems are marked by a concern for fairness and equality they are often seen as embodying egalitarianism, which is a broad term referring to the pursuit of equality and/or equity in public provision. Egalitarianism can take a number of forms depending on how equality is understood. At one extreme, this might involve the strict maxim that everyone should be allotted equal measures of public resources irrespective of their circumstances. More commonly in health care, egalitarianism is linked to levels of need, with the worse off receiving priority in the pursuit of broader equality of health and well-being. Egalitarianism is most common in health care systems characterised by a strong sense of collectivity and solidarity, in which the needs of the whole take precedence over the specific requirements of the individual. The NHS commitment to a comprehensive service, available to all and free at the point of delivery, is quintessentially egalitarian in tone, hinging as it does on a collective commitment to shared values and equal status regardless of personal wealth and/or other individual characteristics. It has been argued that equality of health is more important than equality in other areas of life (such as income and wealth) as poor health reduces more profoundly the scope for full human agency (Anand, 2000).

As with all single principles, egalitarianism has its limitations and, in practice, concern for equality is often tempered by other considerations. For example, a situation where everyone is unwell may be more equitable but less preferable than a situation where some people enjoy good health. Equality must therefore be balanced against the need to consider the requirements of a whole community or population. Identifying measures of equality is also problematic, as we will see in debates described later between those advocating a disease severity approach and those in favour of a 'fair innings' model. What is clear is that if we wish to give priority to those worse off, we must first set parameters of how we will measure this (Nord, 2005).

Individualism

In recent decades, individualism has emerged as an increasingly powerful ethical principle shaping attitudes to health care, to the extent that egalitarian principles have become challenged and/or diluted in health policy and organisation. As we have seen, the clinical profession in the UK and elsewhere has founded much of its ethical codes on a commitment to the individual patient and this has been at odds with the egalitarian codes of the broader system. Policies and reforms designed to promote patient choice in the consumption of health care resources are a reflection of this shift in perspective. If egalitarianism is aligned to a collectivist political ideology, the focus on individual rights and choice is most attuned to modern political liberalism, and the belief that the sovereignty of the patient-consumer trumps considerations of equity and fairness in the allocation of resources.

The individualist perspective raises important ethical questions about the relative weight afforded to the demands of populations and individuals. The rise of consumerism has given birth to a new, more demanding and more articulate patient with greater awareness of their rights and entitlements. However, this development has been uneven and still reflects patterns of inclusion and inequality so that not all patient groups are equally heard or responded to. Is it ethical to allow this 'marketisation' of the public sector to flourish when disparities in health and well-being profiles remain pronounced? On the other hand, how plausible or ethical is it to subject individual service users to the strictures of collective service models when, for example, they are willing and able to pay for additional health services (Øvretveit, 1997)? These debates have recently been played out through the Richards review of access to NHS treatment in which top-up fees were rejected on grounds including considerations of equity (Appleby and Maybin, 2008).

Utilitarianism

Much of the recent drive towards evidence-based priority setting in health care draws on the ethical principle of utilitarianism, which promotes the 'greatest happiness of the greatest number'. In health care, the notion of happiness (or 'utility') has been translated into health maximisation by health economists such as Alan Williams, who argues that: 'In health care, "doing good" means improving people's life expectancy and the quality of their life' (Williams, 1998, p 29). From this perspective, the success or otherwise of priority setting is determined by the *consequences* of the decisions made, and this is measured (at least primarily) in terms of population health gain. Given the realities of scarcity, *efficiency* – achieving the maximum benefit from a given resource – therefore becomes a key utilitarian principle. It is the focus on maximisation of overall population health that distinguishes utilitarian approaches to priority setting from the egalitarian concern with equal distribution, although both approaches are consequentialist and, therefore, arguably capable of being combined (Olsen, 1997).

The utilitarian approach to priority setting hinges on consensus over the fundamental aims of health care, and it is when such consensus is not reached (eg in relation to the importance of health maximisation) that this rational, consequentialist model breaks down. Because health care decision-making is more often than not marked by multiple (and sometimes competing) goals, critics have rejected the strict utilitarian approach as inappropriate (Coast, 2004). However, the influence of the health economics approach has continued to spread in the work of national bodies such as NICE (through its technology appraisals programme), although adoption by local decision-makers remains comparatively rare (Williams and Bryan, 2007a). A more detailed assessment of a utilitarian, evidence-based approach to priority setting is provided in Chapter Four.

Communitarianism

As with egalitarianism, individualism and utilitarianism, the concept of communitarianism contains a variety of formulations and perspectives. Overall, the communitarian position is distinctive in its focus on *procedural* rather than *substantive* justice. From this perspective, the aims of public provision (such as health care) must be established in a process of dialogue with the citizens of the society served. Therefore, in the words of Weale (1995, p 838), allocation of resources 'should depend upon the opinion and expressed preferences of citizens, as aggregated through political process'. These processes will not only help to identify the value-mission of health care, but are also considered valuable inasmuch as they strengthen and reinforce the social contract between state and civic society. This public engagement is very different from engagement with patients and other groups with a stake in the outcome of a particular resource allocation decision as citizen engagement necessarily proceeds under the 'veil of ignorance' (Rawls, 1971) in which we are asked to envisage the type of society (and therefore the type of public services) we wish to bring about, without knowing *who we will be in that society* (Hope, 2001). In Chapter Three we explore in more detail methods for conducting citizen engagement.

Communitarianism has been proposed as a model for priority setting by commentators such as Gavin Mooney (1998), who argue that decisions based solely on measures of need or capacity to benefit fail to engage with the broader social values that shape attitudes to and expectations of health care. In this context, the role of the priority setter is to facilitate such engagement. In the words of Chadwick (1998, p 45): 'the communitarian manager ... seeks to elucidate the communitarian consensus on values to aid him or her in making allocation decisions'. However, communitarianism also has its challenges, for example, the need to educate citizens sufficiently to engage in informed deliberation without this becoming manipulative and suppressive of genuine value differences where these exist.

Just deserts

There are a number of values that might emerge as being important to citizens when drawing up the rules of engagement for priority setting. The notion of desert extends the individualist principle of personal responsibility for health and has a number of potential implications for resource allocation. From a just deserts point of view, it becomes legitimate to de-prioritise individuals whose personal behaviour contributes to their poor health – for example, through smoking, excessive alcohol consumption and/or lack of exercise. The notion of holding people responsible for their behaviour in this way has received some empirical support (Williams, 1992; Dolan and Tsuzhiya, 2009; Michailakis and Schirmer, 2010) and can increasingly be seen in current policy and media rhetoric (eg *Times Online*, 2008). A corollary of the desert principle is the notion of 'getting back what you put in' whereby the extent of people's contribution (eg via tax or social insurance payments) should be a factor in determining levels of access. This is a controversial topic and the just deserts approach attracts vehement criticism from those who consider it to be at best arbitrary (How should we decide which characteristics and behaviours disqualify us from access to care?) and at worst discriminatory, as the disqualifying behaviours commonly cited are more usually prevalent in lower-income, disadvantaged social groups. The just deserts approach is also questionable in its assumptions about human agency and autonomy, for example, the belief that alcoholism is a voluntary behaviour (Caplan, 1994). Furthermore, the potential for social division in the demarcation of the 'social worth' of individuals, based on character traits, also needs to be taken into account in the thorny terrain of priority setting (Øvretveit, 1997).

Rule of rescue

Another ethical imperative that is frequently evoked in relation to health care is the 'rule of rescue', which has been defined as the imperative to attempt to save lives however unlikely the chances of success (Dworkin, 2000). The rule of rescue has been advocated as a principle to inform priority setting in situations where lives are at risk and interventions exist that might prevent death (see eg Jonsen, 1986). Although the notion is linked to the imperative to account for disease severity (discussed later) it is distinct from this in both its tendency to be invoked in relation to *identifiable* individuals and also the extra importance implied by the presence of death in the equation (Singer and Mapa, 1998) so that even treatments that might not save lives – such as care for the terminally ill – are given extra priority (Hope, 2001). Those who argue for the importance of the rule of rescue emphasise both the likelihood that it will only apply in a relatively small number of cases and the additional symbolic value of life-saving. In the words of McKie and Richardson (2003, p 2413): 'people obtain benefit from the belief that they are living in a caring and humane society, and … the observation of heroic attempts to save life reinforces this'.

However, this concept has been criticised as vague and unspecified and its tendency to be invoked in relation to identifiable individuals has led to criticism that rule of rescue scenarios are often contrived by forces such as the media at the expense of both broader population health considerations and less well-publicised individual cases (MacKenzie et al, 2008; Schöne-Seifert, 2009). This 'popularism' weakens the claim to fairness that, it is argued, should be a prerequisite of priority setting. It is on grounds of perceived unfairness (and opportunity cost) that the NICE Citizens Council decided against incorporation of the rule of rescue into its decision-making (NICE, 2006), and it is broadly accepted that, overall, while reflecting important ethical considerations, the rule of rescue should not be operated without due regard to other social values (Cookson et al, 2008).

Disease severity

A related principle that has been brought to bear on the ethical debates around priority setting is that of severity of illness. Erik Nord (2005, p 258) describes this principle thus: 'The basic hypothesis of the severity approach is that the societal value (appreciation) of a health improvement of a given size is greater the greater the severity of the patient's initial condition'.

This hypothesis holds that not all medical needs are equal and that it is morally justified to treat those in greatest need ahead of those who enjoy greater health. So, for example, cancer treatment has a greater claim to urgency than does treatment for acne, irrespective of the measureable benefits of each. However, the notion of disease severity is subject to varying interpretations and requires adjudication between the claims of, for example, degenerative long-term conditions and short-term but potentially fatal illness (Holm, 1998). And, as with the rule of rescue, there remains a requirement to maintain or improve the health of the better off – at what point do we consider aggregation of modest benefits to the many to outweigh greater benefits to the few?

Linked to both the rule of rescue and disease severity is the issue of rare and very rare conditions and whether rationing responses (ie 'orphan-drug' policy) should make allowances for these treatments when they exceed usual costs. The validity of condition prevalence as an ethical consideration is also disputed in the literature (McCabe et al, 2005).

Fair innings

Over the years, numerous commentators have argued that age should be taken into account when drawing up the design rules for priority setting (eg Callahan, 1988; Daniels, 1990) and, with equal frequency, these claims have been disputed (Evans, 1997). The most sustained case made for age-based rationing in recent times has been formulated by Alan Williams (1997). His 'fair innings' model holds that resources should be deployed so as to achieve the most equal distribution of healthy years across a population. This implies that patient groups become less of a priority when they exceed (or are projected to exceed) this fair innings. This approach differs from the disease severity model in that it takes into account the whole lifespan (and in his analysis Williams includes quality of life) rather than just current and future prognosis.

Needless to say, the 'fair innings' model is both controversial and contested. Critics claim that it contravenes human rights and provides a justification for age-based discrimination. Williams (1997) himself acknowledges the need to secure broad societal support for such an approach to priority setting. There are also question marks over the compatibility of the fair innings model with a concern for severity of illness (Nord, 2005). Certainly, it seems unlikely that a unilateral adoption of age-based rationing could be supported without further exploration of both social values and the legal implications. One avenue of possible compromise would be an approach in which life-extending treatments are targeted at younger populations, but palliative and other quality-of-life treatments are made equally available to all.

Learning exercise 2.1: Understanding ethical principles

The following propositions raise ethical issues about the distribution of scarce health care resources. What ethical principles are at play and what would be the responses of egalitarians, libertarians, utilitarians and communitarians?

Interventions that promise to improve the health, well-being and life chances of the young should receive a higher priority than equivalent interventions aimed at the elderly (classed as over 70 years of age).

Smokers who do not commit to undergoing cessation treatment should receive lower priority in the allocation of expensive surgical procedures.

A community hospital with an accident and emergency department should be downgraded/closed on the grounds that it is an inefficient use of resources and potentially unsafe. There is a strong current of local opinion in favour of keeping the hospital open.

The ethical maze of priority setting

Since as early as 1979, rationing has been portrayed as akin to juggling, where success is defined by the extent to which multiple balls can be kept in the air at any one time (Calabresi and Bobbitt, 1979). Although all public-sector resource allocation is ultimately justified by contribution to the public good, health care systems exhibit a confusion of moral values that renders the identification of a coherent guiding ethical framework problematic. What is clear is that not all ethical principles can be pursued simultaneously, at least not to equal extents. This has led to dispute over the relative merits of ethical standpoints and to the development of hybrid approaches. These latter include: subsidiarity, whereby egalitarianism is proposed for some conditions and the rule of rescue for others, for example; or fair chance weighted lotteries that incorporate equity adjustments into a 'first-out-the-hat' overall model (Coast et al, 1996). As Table 2.1 shows, one can observe examples of each of the main ethical precepts currently in the NHS and this goes some way towards explaining why the challenge of priority setting is so great. Resolving this confusion is likely to be difficult and much hinges on

Table 2.1: Examples of ethical principles in the NHS

Egalitarianism	Embodied in the principle that everyone in society will receive equitable access to health care services in a system funded primarily out of general taxation.
Individualism	Reflected in an increased focus on importance of patient choice as a desired end and consumerism as a driver of quality improvement in services.
Utilitarianism	Embodied in the phrase 'adding years to life and life to years' and central to the cost-effectiveness agenda promoted by NICE.
Communitarianism	Reflected in the (limited) emphasis placed on public involvement in the NHS Constitution, NICE, commissioning and other areas of activity.

greater understanding of societal values. We therefore add our voices to the call for greater empirical investigation of values in relation to health care (Ryynanen et al, 1999; Gallego et al, 2007) and the importance of empirical ethics more generally (Richardson, 2002). These themes are returned to in Chapter Three.

Replacing principles with process

Unfortunately those implementing priority setting and resource allocation cannot wait for such ethical clarity to be attained (if indeed this is possible). Holm (1998, p 1001) summarises the predicament:

> If our priorities cannot be directly legitimised as the rational results of following rational rules, what should we then do? We have to make decisions in some way, and we also have to be able to defend them publicly.

He goes on to call for a 'second phase' of priority setting in which principalism is replaced by a concern to establish fair decision-making *processes*. This is supported by evidence which suggests that trust in decision processes is as important as distributional outcomes (Gilson, 2003). Daniels and Sabin (2008, p 4) argue that: 'In the absence of a broadly accepted consensus on principles for fair distribution, the problem of fair allocation becomes one of procedural justice.' Their accountability for reasonableness (A4R) framework has emerged as a leading model of process-based health care decision-making. A4R is made up of four criteria by which the strength of decisions (and the processes they follow) can be measured. The first of these is the *publicity* condition, which holds that decisions taken over the allocation of health care resources should be made accessible to the public. Although this may seem uncontroversial, if adopted fully, the condition disallows implicit rationing and exposes decision-makers to attack – whether from the public or the media – in cases where unpopular determinations are reached. The second condition is that of *relevance* and holds that decisions should be influenced by evidence that fair-minded people would consider relevant so that determinations reached are based on reasonable considerations. The *appeals* condition holds that there must be mechanisms for challenge and review of decisions reached and for resolving any resulting disputes. This presupposes that those implicated in or affected by a decision have a clear understanding of its basis and subscribe to the process of decision review. Finally, the *enforcement* condition requires there to be effective mechanisms for ensuring the other three conditions are implemented and regulated. In other words, it puts teeth into the overall framework.

By instituting a formal process, A4R is designed to improve the consistency of decision-making in a way that is analogous to the development of legal case law. Daniels and Sabin (2008) argue that, over time, a form of institutionalist reflective equilibrium will be achieved in which revisions to what are considered reasonable drivers of decisions take place only in response to important new developments or external changes, and then only after careful deliberation. The

A4R framework is not only concerned with the quality and coherence of the decision-making process, but also with communitarian notions of engagement, democracy and legitimacy. Daniels and Sabin argue that neither philosophical nor empirical foundations are sufficient to provide legitimacy for rationing decisions as this can only be achieved through a process of engagement with stakeholders and the public.

Although A4R has become a popular and useful tool for priority setters in a range of contexts, it has also been criticised. The most contentious aspect of the framework has proved to be the relevance condition. Whilst, at the extremes, it may be possible (as well as useful) to rule out irrelevant perspectives and factors from consideration, there is likely to be disagreement in some areas. For Daniels and Sabin (2008), reasonable considerations are those that are aligned to the promotion of equal opportunity (ie by allocating according to the extent of impairment) and this disqualifies reasoning based on religious world views that do not take a whole-population perspective. However, critics such as Friedman (2008, p 109) argue that these distinctions break down under scrutiny and that 'there is no clear and non-controversial way to draw the line demarcating "bad" (non-public) religious reasons from "good" (public) philosophical ones' and that, therefore, the relevance condition ought not to be implemented. Writing in a different context, Young (2000, p 108) offers a warning against complacent assumptions about what is or is not a reasonable perspective:

> Under circumstances of structural and economic inequality, the relative power of some groups often allows them to dominate the definition of the common good in ways compatible with their experience, perspective and priorities. A common consequence of social privilege is the ability of a group to convert its perspective in some issues into authoritative knowledge without being challenged by those who have reason to see things differently.

In acknowledgement of the importance of inequality in decision-making, Gibson et al (2005) propose a fifth condition of 'empowerment', which refers to the imperative to minimise power differences between participants.

Other commentators remain well disposed to the A4R framework – especially its three process-based conditions – whilst acknowledging variation in what is considered reasonable or fair across contexts (Kapiriri et al, 2009). Hasman and Holm (2005, p 272) conclude that 'Legitimation through process, and not directly through the notion of fairness, is the most important component of the A4R framework.'

Further criticism of A4R relates to the extent to which adherence to its conditions actually confers legitimacy on the subsequent rationing of services. Kapiriri et al (2009), for example, note that levels of public involvement may need to be greater than is advocated by Daniels and Sabin. Friedman (2008, p 103) concurs, arguing: 'The Publicity and Revision/Appeals Conditions permit an insufficient amount of public involvement to support claims of democratic legitimacy on procedural grounds'. Irrespective of these debates, A4R and the pursuit of fair process is an important development in understanding priority setting in health care, and one that provides practical support for decision-makers. This is especially so given the increasingly ambivalent role played by legal institutions in health care resource allocation. Although the threat of legal challenge has always loomed over those withholding treatment (Hope, 2001), the role of the courts within the UK has appeared to shift in recent times. Newdick and Derrett (2006) distinguish between negative and positive rights of individuals and the role of the courts in protecting these. Negative rights protect the freedoms of individuals (eg to refuse consent for treatment on grounds of self-determination), whereas positive rights relate to the individual's claim to be allowed to access services. These positive rights are more difficult for legal bodies to adjudicate because of the strain on public resources, and the relative lack of expertise possessed by the courts in population-based decision-making. However, recent cases indicate a trend towards legal support for the rights-based claims of individuals to treatment access. Process models such as A4R may help provide a counterweight to unrealistic claims to substantive rights through demonstration that fair and consistent decision processes have been followed.

> ## Box 2.1: Guide rules for considerations of ethics in priority setting
>
> 1. Understand and discuss the ethical principles that can and/or should underpin priority-setting decisions.
> 2. In particular, be aware of the egalitarian, individualist (or libertarian), communitarian and utilitarian perspectives on how resources should be allocated.
> 3. Develop policy stances in relation to personal responsibility, the rule of rescue, disease severity and the fair innings principles, and the weight attached to these in resource allocation decisions.
> 4. Implement processes that meet the criteria described in the accountability for reasonableness framework.

Chapter summary

Those involved in the allocation of scarce resources in health care face a number of ethical challenges as all principle-based decision criteria are open to legitimate challenge, and there remains an absence of an agreed, single principle by which priority-setting decisions can be judged. For example, the aim of maximising health gain for a population can run counter to the promotion of equal access and reducing health inequalities. To these imperatives can be added notions of: fairness, accountability, the rule of rescue, disease severity and choice. This chapter has described the main ethical principles underpinning health care systems and the challenge this multiplicity poses to resource allocators seeking to adopt explicit approaches to priority setting. Ethical frameworks designed to help decision-makers reconcile these tensions (such as A4R) can help to provide practical strategies for navigating this complexity. However, A4R does not replace the need for engagement at the level of ethical principles and does not obviate the requirement for difficult deliberations to be conducted between parties who disagree about how resources should be allocated. The following chapters tackle these difficulties through attention to public involvement, evidence, politics and leadership.

Learning exercise 2.2: Applying accountability for reasonableness

Decisions over the allocation of public resources can be measured according to the four conditions of A4R. Consider a decision-making process that you have been involved with and how well it performs in terms of publicity, relevance, appeals and enforcement.

THREE

Public participation in priority setting

Key points covered in Chapter Three

- There are a range of reasons to involve the public in priority-setting processes and a number of mechanisms for carrying this out. Selection of approach should reflect overall aims of the involvement programme.
- Participation in priority setting is best suited to deliberative citizen engagement using techniques such as citizens' juries, consensus conferences and deliberative polling. These approaches each have strengths and weaknesses and can be used in combination.
- Deliberative group methods are specifically designed to tackle polarising and potentially divisive topics and decisions.
- Deliberative approaches are intended to inform preferences as well as capture them, and often result in participants changing their views.
- Public engagement does not provide a panacea for the problems of priority setting and there are limitations relating to: resource constraints; incentivising participation; the representativeness of participants; issues of power and manipulation; trust deficits; and tokenism.

Introduction

In the field of priority setting, lines of enquiry, debate and analysis invariably arrive at a realisation of the need to involve the public. There are a number of reasons why this is the case. As we have seen, resource allocation in health care has yet to operate from a foundation of ethical clarity and consensus, and, indeed, may never succeed in doing so. Furthermore, health care resource allocation remains highly politicised and subject to the sectional agendas of interest groups (discussed further in Chapter Six). For these reasons, commentators repeatedly assert the dependence of future progress on our ability to identify the rationing priorities of the public. Ultimately, the argument goes, only *citizens* can furnish decision-makers with a valid account of the public good that resource allocation should support. As agents of this broader constituency, rationers must therefore be aware of (and in tune with) social values and the expectations society holds of its health care system. Rather than being a counterweight to citizen priorities, evidence, expertise and stakeholder input should thus be the servant of the democratically expressed will of the public (Mooney, 1998).

As well as being a prerequisite of 'successful' decision-making, public involvement also promises to enhance the civic and democratic fabric of society through the promotion of active citizenship – augmenting the passive citizenship of traditional liberal democracy (Smith and Wales, 2000). These dual imperatives are enshrined in the Council of Europe's assertion of the democratic importance of citizen involvement in determining the goals of health care systems (Council of Europe, 2000). Closer to home, National Health Service (NHS) policy has for some time now cited the importance of patient, consumer and public involvement, albeit without substantive consideration of these in relation to priority setting (Florin and Dixon, 2004; Thompson, 2007; Forster and Gabe, 2008). Perhaps surprisingly, given the frequency with which public participation is prescribed, citizens remain largely outside of health system decision-making structures and processes across the developed world (Callaghan and Wistow, 2006; Vergel and Ferguson, 2006; Menon et al, 2007; Sabik and Lie, 2008). In this chapter, the evidence base on public participation in priority setting is summarised and the notion of *deliberative* engagement is explained in detail. The chapter then covers a series of key themes and recommendations for those seeking to engage their publics in priority-setting decisions.

Terminology

The public involvement literature is marked by definitional complexity, not least with respect to the terms 'public' and 'involvement' themselves. Adapting Parry et al (1992, p 16, cited in Litva et al, 2002, p 1826), we propose the following definition of involvement:

> Taking part in the process of formulation, passage, and implementation of public policies [through] action by citizens which is aimed at influencing decisions which are, in most cases, ultimately taken by public representatives and officials.

This definition contains a number of important elements. First, it recognises that policies – for example, with respect to investment in specific health care interventions – can be shaped and influenced at multiple stages, and, indeed, many policies look quite different from their initial formulation by the time they are implemented. Second, the emphasis is on *citizens* – as opposed to patients, consumers and stakeholders. The importance of this distinction is explored later. Finally, the definition refers to influence over decisions that are formally the jurisdiction of public-sector professionals and representatives. Therefore, it draws our attention to the role played by the public in both democratic and administrative functions of public-sector decision-making. This requires us to consider the relationship between citizens and agents of the state (ie elected and appointed public-sector managers and decision-makers) and how authority and influence should be distributed between these.

Despite these important aspects, Parry et al's definition remains broad in scope and does not, for example, make distinctions based on either *extent* or *type* of involvement. Given that there are numerous involvement mechanisms to choose from – based on a scoping review of the published literature, Mitton et al (2009) identified 405 techniques – it is perhaps helpful to provide further specification and subdivision of involvement strategies. To this end, Rowe and Frewer (2005) distinguish between *communicative, consultative* and *participative* forms. The key point of interest here is that only the interventions categorised as participative involve dialogue. Communication involves transferring information *to* (as opposed to *from*) the public, and consultation involves extracting data on public opinion (eg through large-scale postal surveys) without providing opportunities for discussion. By contrast, participative involvement requires a more substantive interaction between citizens and decision-makers. It has been argued that public involvement within health care in general (and the NHS in particular) has tended to adopt a communication and consultation model with limited opportunities for participation (Callaghan and Wistow, 2006). As well as distinguishing participation from other forms of involvement, the work of Arnstein (1969) and others has helped to map the levels or *extent* of involvement, and to understand the implications of this for the distribution of power between decision-makers and the public (see Figure 3.1). Arnstein maps a spectrum of engagement ranging from manipulation, through tokenism, to models that involve genuine citizen power over decision-making.

All too often, discussions of involvement (or participation) also fall short of full clarity over what is meant by the 'public'. Crucially, there is a need for separation of public involvement – which refers to citizens – and other forms of involvement (eg patient, consumer or stakeholder). In Chapter Six, we discuss the role of stakeholders and interest groups in priority setting and clearly there is a strong argument for seeking the input of the health care user and consumer when planning health services. However, whilst patient and consumer involvement foregrounds individual rights, experiences and preferences, *public* involvement is primarily a collective model of engagement. So whereas patient and service-user groups may play a key role in pathway design and service evaluation, they are not typically well suited for involvement in questions relating to the public good (Gilbert, 2007), and strategies such as the exercising of 'choice' and 'exit' are not applicable to citizen participation in population health decisions (Callaghan and Wistow, 2006).

Lomas (1997) identifies three main characterisations of the citizen as an active contributor to the rationing process:

1. The citizen-taxpayer concerned with how services are financed.
2. The citizen-collective decision-maker concerned with the range of services available.
3. The citizen-patient concerned with how the health needs of patients (in general) will be met.

Figure 3.1: Arnstein's ladder of involvement

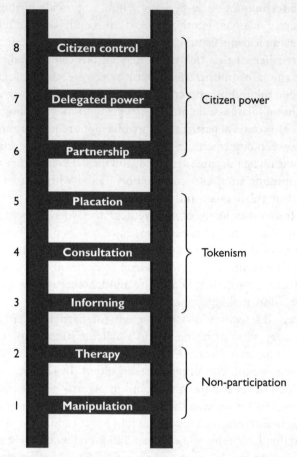

Source: Arnstein (1969)

Each of these roles is underpinned by the principle of depersonalisation. In other words, the participant is required to consider benefits to a *population* rather than advancing his or her own concerns. Lomas also identifies three types of decisions into which public input might be sought:

1. The allocation of funds to health (as opposed to other sectors and service areas).
2. The allocation of funds to specific health services and programmes.
3. The allocation of funds and resources to patient populations and groups.

To these, Mullen (1999) adds two further opportunities for public input into priority setting:

1. Decisions over the location of service provision (eg local or central, acute or community).

2. Decisions over treatment for individual patients (eg through public input into decision criteria).

Another important distinction in approaches to citizen participation is between the collection of *individual* and *collective* views. Both can be administered in such a way as to facilitate deliberation.

These insights indicate that public involvement in priority setting can take a variety of forms and applications, and deciding which approach to take requires clarity in relation to the aims and objectives of the involvement enterprise. Arguably, however, involvement policies as set down by health ministries have been less than clear on the purposes these are intended to advance. In other words, public involvement has been deemed a 'good thing' without an account of why this might be the case.

Why involve the public in priority setting?

The benefits attributed to public involvement in priority setting fall into three broad categories: instrumental, political and educative.

Instrumental benefits

By helping to identify and advance the intended goals of health care, public input can improve the quality, consistency and appropriateness of resource allocation. In particular, public involvement is seen as key to resolving the ethical dilemmas examined in Chapter Two, based on the assumption that without reliable information on citizen preferences it is impossible to establish an ethical basis from which to distribute scarce health care resources. This argument is instrumentalist in the sense that it focuses on the *ends* brought about by involvement (ie better decisions). Instrumental approaches to public involvement inform the quantitative preference-elicitation techniques discussed in Chapter Four as well as population surveys such as those carried out by Heginbotham (1993) and Bowling (1996).

Political benefits

It is often argued that the NHS suffers from a 'democratic deficit' resulting from the limited avenues for local democratic input into its decision-making structures and the perception that a centralist bureaucracy remains dominant (Tritter and McCallum, 2006). From this point of view, the participation of citizens in priority setting has intrinsic value in its contribution to democratic accountability. This recalls the communitarian principle described in Chapter Two and the contention that engagement can help to bind disparate groups together through the collective expression of political or civic identity (Litva et al, 2002). The democratic deficit – and the broader erosion of trust in mainstream political processes – requires this new form of engagement to embrace the shift from *representative* to *deliberative* democracy through greater involvement of stakeholders in decision-making (Barnes et al, 2007). For these political (or communitarian) benefits to be felt, public involvement must be *participative*, thereby fostering active citizenship and promoting deliberative democracy (Waite and Nolte, 2006).

Educative benefits

The third area of support for public involvement lies in the presumed educational benefits accrued to citizens. Thus, advocates argue that in an explicit priority-setting process, public engagement can help to provide the informed deliberation required for the unpalatable realities of rationing to be understood and accepted (Mooney, 1998). This is especially pertinent in relation to the NHS as there is an apparent 'delivery paradox' whereby observable improvements in health system performance run ahead of public perceptions, so that trust in the institutions of health care erodes even as those institutions improve (Blaug et al, 2006). It has been argued that governments have fostered unrealistic expectations of what health care systems can deliver without acknowledgement of the subsequent difficulties this presents to decision-makers. This was acknowledged by Sir Ian Kennedy (cited in Newdick and Derrett, 2006, p 158) when he argued: 'the public has been led to believe that the NHS could meet their legitimate needs, whereas it is patently clear that it could not'. Research provides some support for this idea of participation as a means of educating the public as to the difficulties of rationing (Dolan et al, 1999; Williams et al, 2011b).

When taken together, these three dimensions – *improving quality*, *enhancing democracy* and *raising awareness* – would suggest that public participation is of significant importance to the priority-setting enterprise. They also imply the need for a deliberative, interactive approach in which pre-held views are examined and challenged, especially where decisions are complex, contested, involve ethical trade-offs and require public support for their implementation. This links to the notion of public engagement as a method for enhancing *social capital* (Tritter and McCallum, 2006, p 163) and the belief that 'a reflective, critical populace is a prerequisite for meaningful social change' (Loughlin, 1998).

Learning exercise 3.1: Involvement from a citizen perspective

Put yourself in the role of citizen and consider the following: What health care resource allocation decisions would you most like to be involved in?; What, if any, health care resource allocation decisions would you prefer not to be involved in?; What would help to incentivise you to be involved?; How would you expect your involvement (and that of other citizens) to impact on resource allocation decisions?; And how would you prefer to be informed of the outcomes of the involvement process?

Participative public involvement methods

Assessing and selecting from the wide array of involvement mechanisms is a challenge for priority setters not just because of the variety of options to choose from, but also because many mechanisms can (and in some cases should) be used in combination. Furthermore, use of nomenclature can vary according to different settings with, for example, the term 'citizens' panel' understood differently in different countries (Rowe and Frewer, 2005). As already argued, the focus here is on deliberative methods as those most likely to facilitate the types of citizen engagement that are considered most useful for priority setting. Excluded from this, therefore, are communication and consultation, as well as the involvement of individuals (eg lay representatives) on decision-making panels and boards otherwise made up of experts and professionals. This latter model – a common feature of many NHS involvement strategies – cannot in itself be expected to deliver the wider benefits attributed to more substantive deliberative engagement programmes (Bruni et al, 2008).

The focus of the remainder of this chapter is therefore on deliberative group methods – citizens' juries, consensus conferences and deliberative polling (Abelson et al, 2003). This is not an exhaustive list, but we would argue that other techniques constitute variations on (rather than departures from) these models. Each incorporates face-to-face interaction with decision-makers, and each can be carried out with uninformed or (more commonly) informed participants (Harrison and Mort, 1998). In each case, deliberation is foregrounded in the pursuit of common understandings and mutual respect, as participants with opposing perspectives enter into dialogue with one another (Gutmann and Thompson, 2004). Deliberative approaches are thus specifically designed to tackle polarising and potentially divisive topics and decisions. The rationale behind deliberative approaches is that rationing decisions are emotive, complex and subject to disagreement, and that it is therefore imperative that participants with a range of views are given the opportunity to share and discuss these in a safe and controlled environment. In all deliberative approaches, therefore, the facilitator or moderator role is extremely important, as is the early establishment of rules of conduct. Deliberative approaches are intended to *inform* preferences as much as to *capture* them, and invariably result in participants changing their views (Paul et al, 2008).

Citizens' juries

The most commonly adopted approach to deliberation is the citizens' jury (Davies et al, 2006). There are variations in their application, but, in the main, citizens' juries adopt the following process:

- A number of between 12 and 25 citizens meet to deliberate on a topic or question over a period of several days.

- Participants are selected randomly or according to specific sampling criteria – that is, to ensure that a spread is included (eg according to age, gender and ethnicity).
- Participants are provided with written information to help inform their discussions.
- Participants hear testimony of 'witnesses' – experts and/or representatives with an interest in the topic – and have an opportunity to question and cross-examine them.
- Participants deliberate over the evidence in small groups and arrive at decisions and/or recommendations with the help of a trained facilitator.
- The final outcomes are formally reported in a written document.

A notable variant of the citizens' jury is the citizens' panel (Abelson et al, 2003), which involves a similar number of participants in similar activities, but which has more permanency: for example, citizens' panel members may continue to meet over longer periods of time to discuss multiple topics. Citizens' juries and panels have been commissioned in the UK at multiple decision levels and in relation to a variety of health-related issues (see eg McIver, 1998).

Consensus conferences

Consensus conferences share some features with citizens' juries, but are designed to facilitate deliberation on issues of a technical or scientific nature (Guston, 1999). Consensus conference processes may vary, but typically involve the following:

- Citizens meet in small groups to discuss scientific or technical issues.
- Facilitated support and advice is provided to enable agreement to be reached by the citizen group on the subject in question.
- A second meeting is held to which experts, the media and the wider public are invited, and where the conclusions and recommendations of the citizen group are presented.
- A collective drawing together of observations and conclusions is undertaken.
- The final outcomes are formally reported in a written document.

The most common function of consensus conferences has been to aid and disseminate medical insights, and they have been used to inform clinical guideline development. However, they have also proved useful in helping to bridge the gap between medicine and the public (Joss and Durant, 1995). In the case of priority setting, consensus conferences might be useful, therefore, in helping to simplify some of the complexities associated with decision-making. Clearly this model is more explicit than the citizens' jury in its concern with consensus-building.

Deliberative polling

Deliberative polling attempts to combine the benefits of quantitative opinion polling with group deliberation (Fishkin, 1991). Luskin et al (2002) explain the distinctive features of the approach:

> An ordinary poll is designed to show what the public actually thinks about some set of issues however little, irreflective, and changeable that may be, and generally is. A Deliberative Poll is designed to show what the public would think about the issues, if it thought more earnestly and had more information about them.

As such, deliberative processes are incorporated into standard polling techniques through follow-up discussion with respondents. The process for carrying this out is as follows:

- A sample of citizens is selected randomly or according to specific criteria.
- The views of those who agree to participate are elicited in relation to the topic of interest views (eg via a survey tool).
- Relevant information and materials are then sent to respondents to help stimulate and develop their views.
- Over a period of several days, participants meet in small groups to discuss the issues. These discussions involve access to experts, representatives and evidence as appropriate.
- The initial data-collection exercise (eg questionnaire) is repeated.
- The outcome of the post-event poll is published and disseminated.

Deliberative polls are similar to the two previous models in that they facilitate face-to-face interaction, involve the use of information materials and rely heavily on facilitation (Mansbridge, 2010). They differ in that they generate *individual* views, albeit ones shaped by group deliberation. Although the intention is to obtain informed preferences, final results are aggregative rather than consensual (Abelson et al, 1995). Given the additional elements and larger scale, deliberative polling is unsurprisingly considerably more expensive to carry out than citizens' juries and consensus conferences.

Box 3.1: The NICE Citizens' Council

NICE's Citizens' Council was established in 2002 as a method for deliberating on the social value trade-offs informing its guidance on access to new technologies. It is made up of 30 members selected to match the population profile of England and Wales in terms of age, gender, ethnicity and socio-economic status. Members 'do not represent any particular section or sector of society, but bring their own personal attitudes, preferences, beliefs and prejudices' (NICE, 2008, pp 8–9). Members must not be health care professionals and each serves a three-year period on the council.

Council meetings are convened to discuss an ethical issue important to NICE work programmes. Meetings are facilitated by an independent organisation and witnesses are cross-examined by council members before conclusions are presented in a report to the NICE board.

Box 3.2: Community involvement in priority setting in NHS County Durham

In 2009, NHS County Durham and Darlington Primary Care Trust (PCT) engaged local citizens in a series of priority-setting simulation events in which participants were asked to take the role of decision-makers, allocating resources to services and patients. Participants were sampled according to purposive and convenience criteria and the events were supported by technology (voting pads) and expert, small-group facilitation.

The primary aims were to understand local public values and also to raise awareness amongst residents of the challenges of population-based decision-making. Dice games were used to introduce elements of chance into the scenarios depicted and opportunities for deliberation and reflection were incorporated throughout.

The instrumental impact of the exercise (ie the impact on actual PCT resource allocation) has yet to be demonstrated. However, participants generally valued and enjoyed the experience and cited considerable educative benefits.

Source: Williams et al (2011b).

Each of these techniques can be combined with other methods of engagement. It is not uncommon, for example, for deliberative priority-setting exercises to also incorporate quantifiable preference–elicitation exercises (Mullen, 1999). These can be useful for measuring, for example, the extent to which attitudes shift during the course of the deliberation. However, for most deliberative exercises, sample sizes are likely to preclude the generation of significant volumes of quantitative data, and there are also some concerns over the validity of data aggregation in this context

(Mullen, 1999). An example of the use of combined quantitative and qualitative approaches can be seen in the methodology of America Speaks (see Box 3.3). The use of communications technology has also opened up the possibility of remote deliberation. Further detail on preference-elicitation techniques is provided in Chapter Four and discussion of communications technology as a means to facilitate deliberation is provided by Coleman and Gøtze (2002).

Box 3.3: America Speaks – a mass approach to public involvement

The America Speaks model of citizen engagement seeks to establish large-scale participation without sacrificing the principles of deliberative engagement. The process begins with an 'issue framing' phase where a policy advisory board and citizens' jury develop topics for deliberation and associated educational materials. Decision-makers are then involved in six complementary public engagement forums in order that commitment to act on results can be secured. The six methods are as follows (adapted from America Speaks, 2004):

- *National 21st-century town meetings* – multiple large-scale forums conducted simultaneously and linked together through interactive video teleconferencing to create a 'National Town Meeting'. Each site uses keypad polling and groupware computers to enable thousands of people to deliberate face to face.
- *Local 21st-century town meetings* – Further forums that engage thousands of people in discussion at a single location, supported by keypad polling and groupware computers.
- *Proxy dialogues* – A television programme that takes viewers through the deliberative process and then solicits their views over the web.
- *Online deliberations* – Small-group dialogue facilitated over the Internet.
- *Community forums* – Smaller, decentralised forums facilitated by local organisations who receive technical assistance and training.
- *Self-facilitated discussions* – Self-facilitated discussions conducted by citizens in their homes and places of work supported by discussion leader kits that include videos and discussion guides.

Assessing deliberative involvement techniques

Although in this chapter we have echoed those who call for routine and substantive public participation in priority setting, the underdeveloped nature of the evidence base on deliberative methods in priority setting would imply that caution is required (Abelson et al, 2003; Rowe and Frewer, 2005; Mitton et al, 2009). The research and evaluation that has been conducted gives grounds for some optimism regarding the instrumental, political and educative benefits, but public engagement falls short of providing a panacea for the problems of priority setting (Abelson et al, 2003; Sabik and Lie, 2008). The main areas of concern for those engaging in such programmes are as follows.

Resources

Deliberative public engagement programmes are costly, time-consuming and complex to design and implement (Abelson et al, 1995). Overall, the expense depends on the numbers involved, extent of information and expertise included, and the number of questions/topics covered. In cases where deliberative engagement is carried out on a large scale, the costs can literally run into millions of pounds (Mitton et al, 2009). Clearly this has implications for those allocating resources to engagement programmes, although, as Bruni et al (2008) note, this should be offset against the time and resources that may be spent addressing subsequent public objections to decisions taken without their involvement. Clearly, consideration should be given to the likely benefits of the engagement exercise, the opportunity cost of carrying it out and the availability of resources to pay for it. It is almost certainly not possible for substantive citizen participation in every resource allocation decision taken. This means that such engagement as is undertaken should serve to inform multiple decisions – for example, through the making of recommendations on general ethical principles and trade-offs – and to cover a suitably broad scale of decision-making functions and target populations. Decisions that concern especially large sums of public money, or which are likely to split public opinion, might also be targeted for citizen involvement. Conversely, participation may be deemed inappropriate in some circumstances. For example, it may be deemed unrealistic and impractical for local priority setters to lead deliberation on matters relating to the direction of national policy.

Incentivising participation

There is considerable dispute within the literature as to whether or not the public are willing to play an active role in priority-setting decisions, with some authors cautiously optimistic (eg McIver, 1998; Wiseman et al, 2003) and others markedly less so (Lomas, 1997; Gallego et al, 2007). It is probably fair to say that much of the drive towards public involvement in priority setting has come from government policy and diktat rather than from a spontaneous groundswell of the public itself (Waite and Nolte, 2006). So to what extent can we assume that if the opportunities for involvement are made available, citizens will take advantage of them? In their study, Litva et al (2002) find that the majority of respondents wished to be involved at the system level of decision-making, approximately half at the programme level and a small minority in terms of decisions over treatment for individual patients. Clearly, those conducting public participation exercises will be required to incentivise involvement without compromising their sampling strategies. Insights from research into the circumstances under which members of the public are likely to be receptive to proposals for participation are important to consider when designing involvement programmes.

Representativeness of public engagement participants

While it is sensible to select participants to reflect characteristics of a broader population, this does not equate to achieving a representative sample. Overall, it is important that sampling strategies are both informed and realistic. Most deliberative approaches are necessarily small scale and therefore do not provide a democratic mandate for action on a scale to match formal political processes. However, this lack of representativeness should not be used as grounds for rejecting the outcomes of deliberative exercises, which should remain an important factor in priority-setting decisions (Davies et al, 2006). Furthermore, through active publicising of recommendations (common in, for example, consensus conferences), deliberative exercises can trigger debate in broader public circles and in the media.

The issue of incentives for involvement is linked to a broader concern with achieving the appropriate sample of participants. As we have seen, participants can be randomly selected from the electoral roll, or else sampling can be purposive – that is, guided by a concern to include a range in terms of gender, ethnicity and so on. However, in either instance there is likely to be significant levels of self-selection as many potential respondents will decline involvement. The effects of this self-selection on deliberations and outcomes are not easy to predict, but one consequence may be that a proportion of participants will have unusually strident or personally felt views on the topic or decision in question. There is also a concern that filtering processes for selection may lead to the over-representation of participants deemed 'appropriate' or acquiescent by decision-makers (Martin, 2008). Klein (1984) identifies an inverse law of participation whereby those least likely (or able) to self-select – so-called 'hard-to-reach' groups – have the most need to do so. The broader public participation literature reinforces the view that initiatives can compound patterns of social exclusion (Barnes et al, 2007). In the case of citizens' panels, which meet over long periods of time, there is also the danger of professionalisation whereby participants become inculcated into a bureaucratic mindset that is at odds with the citizen perspective they are intended to provide.

These are not easy problems to resolve, especially in situations where recruitment to deliberative programmes is difficult to incentivise. However, concerns over representativeness should not be allowed to derail deliberative exercises entirely. After all, public engagement of this type is intended as a form of micro-democracy, designed to augment rather than replace wider democratic processes (Parkinson, 2004). With the partial exception of deliberative polling, mass participation is not facilitated by deliberative approaches (Mansbridge, 2010). There are sound reasons for this, not least the importance of operating on a small scale in the deliberative phase (Smith and Wales, 2000). Indeed, it is unrealistic to expect any sample of 25 or fewer people to be representative of a broader population, however stringent the sampling criteria and recruitment process. Rather, the object is to achieve a profile of participants that is a reasonable approximation of a broader population. The public is invariably characterised by a level of heterogeneity that cannot be matched in such a small sample and it is therefore ill-advised to talk about the public in ways that imply a unified body of experience and/or opinion (Contandripoulos et al, 2004).

Governance and expertise

As noted earlier in the chapter, the exclusion of the public from priority setting is notable given the frequency with which it is advocated within the literature. In Chapter Six, we discuss the impact on resource allocation decisions of the broader organisational and institutional context and this will also influence the extent to which decision-makers are disposed to conducting meaningful and substantive public participation. This suggests the importance of encouraging institutional cultures and governance networks that embrace an outward-facing, inclusive model of decision-making. From this perspective, the public should form a key part of the broader inter-organisational networks present in health care (Callaghan and Wistow, 2006). And rather than being occasional and episodic, public involvement exercises should be conducted as part of an ongoing dialogue – so-called 'fishbowl planning' (Berry et al, 1984). This acknowledges that public preferences 'are not fixed and stable, but are instead adaptive to a wide range of factors' and therefore will shift and change over time (Goodin and Pettit, 2006, p 127).

The exclusion of the public from priority setting often reflects a belief that citizens lack the requisite skills to contribute to complex resource allocation decisions. This rational model of health care decision-making tends to privilege evidence and expertise over involvement and debate (Callaghan and Wistow, 2006). Although the complexity of rationing decisions can be an impediment to participation (Abelson et al, 1995), the more common experience is positive (see eg Gold, 2005). As Coote and Lenaghan (1997, pp 88–9) observe in relation to a citizens' jury: 'we were deeply impressed – as were most other observers – with the level of competence with which jurors tackled their task'. However, there remains an unequal distribution of power in local health governance systems and this can militate against substantive citizen participation (Jessop, 2003). Such barriers are not easily overcome, but a first step is recognition of the role played by institutions and those powerful within them in excluding lay and other stakeholder involvement in policy (Dryzek, 2001).

Consensus and manipulation

We have seen that one of the possible benefits of deliberation is to increase mutual understanding and the likelihood of forming a consensus on controversial topics (Gutmann and Thompson, 2004). However, this consensus-seeking should not be pursued at the cost of respect for diversity and recognition of genuine differences where these exist. The public report having at times felt manipulated in deliberative events (Abelson et al, 1995) and it is important, therefore, not to assume unanimity is achievable and to build space for disagreement into the deliberative process. The facilitator's role is crucial in this respect as they seek to avoid censure of necessarily divergent participatory approaches and styles, while at the same time ensuring adherence to agreed rules of conduct.

As with the issue of governance and expertise, this barrier derives from the relations of power surrounding deliberative exercises and decision-making more generally. For the political (ie democratic) benefits of involvement to be felt, there is a requirement for equality of participation and this extends to the selection of topics for deliberation. It has been argued that public involvement at local levels can exacerbate a disproportionate focus on high-profile or sensationalised issues over those that are less well known but equally important (Iredale and Longley, 1999). Similarly, a populist approach to topic selection may obscure the needs and concerns of minority population groups and or less glamorised services (Waite and Nolte, 2006). To combat this, some advocate the setting up of a steering group comprising key stakeholders' interest groups to set the questions discussed by participants (Smith and Wales, 2000).

Trust

Deliberation is intended to facilitate the build-up of trust and respect between citizens and decision-makers. Gilson (2003, p 1461) describes the process as follows:

> If undertaken freely and openly, the process of communication and dialogue with others requires us to confront the mis-matches between our own beliefs and those of others, enabling self-reflection and learning. Such discourse can not only encourage mutual respect, but also generate the mechanisms, such as shared understanding, persuasion, promises, that align self-interest with the collective interest and so build trust.

However, priority setting takes place against the backdrop of increasing public disillusionment with mainstream politics and a long-term decline in political participation (Forster and Gabe, 2008). Furthermore, high-profile cases of rationing have often resulted in public-sector managers being the target of considerable media and public opprobrium. It is difficult to establish relationships of trust in this context and decision-makers may fear public backlash if decisions are opened up to genuine public debate.

Such concerns may be behind what Martin (2008, p 1757) refers to as a 'widely observed reluctance on the part of health professionals and managers to engage with the public and put into practice the outputs of public involvement processes'. However, there are grounds to believe that the public accept the need for priority setting. For example, government consultation on the NHS Constitution acknowledged that people realise the need for health care provision for individuals to be offset against the need to distribute resources fairly across communities (Newdick and Derrett, 2006). This illustrates the two-way nature of the public participation contract, with public administrator confidence in the constituencies they serve (manifest as a willingness to share decision-making) a precondition of a mutually trusting relationship (Yang, 2005). As already noted, this confidence on the part of decision-makers in health care is often not evident in practice. Indeed, the public administrators' traditional reluctance to forgo autonomy and discretionary authority has led some to ask 'why would anyone with power want to share it?' (Hogg, 2007, p 131). However, the need to secure legitimacy for rationing decisions in health care offers a potentially powerful incentive to do just that. The deliberative process creates opportunities for testing the rationale for decisions. This enables health organisations to develop decision-making that can stand up to public and media scrutiny, thereby enhancing accountability and 'defendability'.

Influencing decisions and outcomes

The use of public engagement as a means to secure support for unpalatable choices over resource allocation has led some to doubt the authenticity of decision-makers' commitment to genuine public participation, claiming that these remain merely a legitimacy device (Harrison and Mort, 1998; Milewa et al, 1999). Support for this claim can be found in the lack of a demonstrable impact of engagement activities on actual resource decisions (Contandripoulos et al, 2004; Mitton et al, 2009). Yang (2005, p 277) argues that 'policy makers tend to ignore the implementation process of participation initiatives, and many frontline administrators do not believe citizens are able to help them with their performance'. This leads to accusations that decision-makers will 'cherry-pick' results that suit them and reject those with inconvenient implications.

Clearly, public participation should make a difference to priority setting if it is worth doing. However, clarity is required over the intended outcomes of deliberative exercises. For example, are the benefits expected to be primarily political and educative, as opposed to instrumental? If so, this should be clearly communicated to potential participants. If the outcomes are intended to be instrumental, a number of questions must be addressed, such as: will results and recommendations be directly consequential or will they be mediated by other considerations? If mediated, how will this process of mediation be conducted and communicated? Although there are well-documented technical difficulties associated with the translation of expressed views and values into decision outcomes (Tenbensel, 2002), there is little by way of practical guidance on how these should be overcome (Mitton et al, 2009). It has been argued that the prevailing rationale for public involvement in the NHS has been to improve the quality of decisions through incorporating a public perspective, but not to submit to fully shared decision-making (Rowe and Shepherd, 2002).

For these reasons it would seem sensible to have plans in place to integrate public values with other decision inputs, and to avoid deliberating on topics that are subject to strong government direction. Priority setters also need to be clear about how the views of the public are incorporated into decision-making processes characterised by interest group contestation and the application of evidence and analysis. In this respect, it is important to avoid the false separation of public participation from other dimensions of priority setting and resource allocation.

Overall, these debates hinge upon broader issues of power in public-sector decision-making, and, as we have seen, the organisations and institutions that make up health care systems reflect an unequal distribution of authority (Parkinson, 2004). Without some genuine transformation of existing power relations, therefore, public participation remains vulnerable to accusations of disingenuousness in the pursuit of political legitimacy (Contandripoulos, 2000).

Based on the discussion presented here, a number of guide rules can be put forward to support those seeking to generate public participation in priority setting and these are set out in Box 3.4.

Learning exercise 3.2: Assessing engagement options

What are the main differences between citizens' panels, consensus conferences and deliberative polling as methods of deliberative engagement?

What are the strengths and weaknesses of each method?

What factors might determine selection of deliberative engagement methods?

Chapter summary

One of the key deficiencies of many existing prescriptions for priority setting is the absence of meaningful engagement of the public in the 'hard choices' involved, and this is reflected in the realities of the resource allocation within health care systems. There are compelling reasons for this gap that relate to the difficulty, cost and risks associated with substantive engagement of the public in the complex and highly charged business of health care rationing. However, it is increasingly accepted that this gap needs to be addressed. This chapter has provided a qualified endorsement of deliberative participation methods based on the instrumental, political and educative benefits this can provide. In instrumental terms, public participation can help to identify the key social value considerations that should guide resource allocation. The political benefits of involvement include not just enhancements to civic engagement, but also potentially increased decision legitimacy. However, legitimacy increases will be short-lived if there is no intention or mechanism to respond to and act upon the views and values expressed. Therefore, it is essential that public participation becomes a genuine driver of decisions. To be successful in this area much depends on the development of trust between administrators and citizens, and to be effective this will need to be a feature of the broader institutional structures and culture. The nature of the governance model adopted by public–sector decision–making bodies will determine the extent and nature of public (as well as other groups') involvement. Therefore, public participation is subject to the effects of political and institutional contexts, and these factors are discussed in more detail in Chapter Six.

Box 3.4: Guide rules for public involvement in priority setting

- *Be clear about the aims of the deliberative exercise*
  When contemplating public participation exercises it should be made clear what the intended benefits are in terms of instrumental, political and educative aspects. These aims will determine what is expected of participants and these should be communicated clearly at the recruitment phase.

- *Set a suitable topic/decision area for deliberation*
  The selection of topics for discussion may reflect a plethora of considerations, including the redundancy of deliberating instrumentally on topics where central guidance is already in place. However, it is also important that the topics chosen are agreed by stakeholders (notably the public itself) to be of importance. The desire to develop consensus on a sensitive or complex topic may also drive topic selection as long as this intention is explicitly declared.

- *Select an appropriate method*
  The choice of deliberative method should flow from the overarching aims of the exercise. For example, expensive and large-scale deliberative polling may be preferred over smaller-scale citizens' juries or panels where broader coverage is required. If a key aim of the exercise is to raise the profile of a particular issue and to stimulate broader debate, consensus conferences may be the most valuable method. However, there is no requirement to slavishly follow prescribed formats: adapting and combining aspects of different models may be important in ensuring compatibility with local aims and contexts.

- *Have a clear sampling frame*
  Irrespective of the approach adopted it is important to have a clear rationale in relation to sampling. Key questions include: what are the selection criteria? Who (if anyone) should be excluded from the exercise (eg current service users and professionals)? Ultimately, the population from which citizens are drawn should be appropriate to the nature and scale of the topic in question.

- *Ensure high-quality facilitation*

  The facilitator role is crucial to successful deliberation. It is also important to set rules of conduct at the outset and to have procedures for assessing educational materials used as well as the selection and input of expert witnesses.

- *Have a clear account of how outcomes will be used*

  It is important that participative exercises are carried out with clear endpoints in mind. This includes an explicit account of how the recommendations reached will impact on decisions. It is also important that the citizen-engagement function is separated from other mechanisms for involvement (ie service user, stakeholder and consumer).

- *Draw on expertise and advice*

  It may be advisable to set up a committee to help devise and implement deliberative exercises, especially those that are large in scale. There are also a range of practical guides and resource repositories for engagement such as those produced by the International Association for Public Participation (see their website at: http://www.iap2.org/).

FOUR

Priority setting and economic evaluation

Key points covered in Chapter Four

- Economic evaluation of health technologies can support priority-setting decisions in a context of resource scarcity.
- Economic evaluation approaches – such as cost–benefit analysis, cost-effectiveness analysis and cost–utility analysis – are underpinned by a number of principles and assumptions that are subject to challenge.
- Summary outcome measures such as Quality Adjusted Life Years and Disability Adjusted Life Years enable broad comparisons of the costs and effects of health care interventions. However, they are based on ethical principles and methodologies that are not universally accepted. Decision-makers should therefore be aware of their strengths and limitations.
- Not all priority setters will have sufficient resources to conduct their own economic evaluations and will therefore be reliant on commissioned or 'off-the-shelf' analyses.
- The existing evidence suggests that economic evaluations are not always compatible with local decision-making contexts in health care.
- Technical approaches such as economic evaluation do not replace the need for engagement and deliberation in priority setting.

Introduction

The shift towards explicit priority setting has led to a growing interest in evidence-based decision-making (Muir Gray, 1997; Niessen et al, 2000; Hewison, 2004). Technical approaches that rely on quantifiable epidemiological, clinical, financial and other data are increasingly used to support and inform decision-making throughout. In particular, there has been a growing interest in decision analysis and predictive modelling with approaches such as economic evaluation becoming markedly more popular since the 1980s (Hauck et al, 2003). This chapter and the next aim to provide a concise, accessible and critical introduction to the main quantitative techniques for supporting health care prioritisation. This chapter focuses on the *economic evaluation* of health care services and interventions, whilst the next chapter introduces some alternative decision-making approaches such as programme budgeting and marginal analysis (PBMA) and multi criteria decision analysis (MCDA). This chapter provides a critical description of the main economic evaluation methods that are used to measure the cost-effectiveness of services. It also explores some of the underpinning theory, details economic resources currently available for priority setters and assesses evidence on the application of economic evaluation in practice. Ultimately, we argue that economic tools may be helpful in supporting priority setting in health care. However, economic evaluation is resource intensive and there are limitations to the use of these techniques in practice, and the skills to support the deployment of these techniques are not always readily available.

Technology coverage decision-making

Health economic analysis provides information on the inputs or costs and the outputs or consequences associated with alternative health care interventions and procedures. In this respect, it is most useful as an aide to *technology coverage* decisions. Decisions to 'cover' technologies (implying that their cost will be reimbursed as part of an insurance package) are taken both in health systems where private insurance is prevalent and in systems dominated by government health insurance programmes. The implication of coverage decisions is that some licensed treatments will be deemed ineffective or inefficient when compared either to treatment alternatives or to some overall standard/threshold. Implications at the policy implementation stage are, therefore, that such treatments are withdrawn from the 'menu' on offer to individual patients and/or patient cohorts. In this respect, technology coverage is a key mechanism for priority setting and the rationing of health care in a context of resource scarcity. Within an English context, technology coverage takes place at a variety of levels including:

- *nationally* through bodies such as NICE and the National Screening Committee;
- at the *local level* through the commissioning activity of Primary Care Trusts (PCTs) and GP-led consortia;
- at the *organisational level* (eg in NHS Trusts through board, directorate and medicines management functions); and
- at the *level of the individual* professional and patient – who is increasingly encouraged to exercise choice, voice and exit in relation to their own health care.

Entry and exit of health care interventions (or 'technologies') from formulary lists can be administered at levels ranging from the organisational (eg the hospital formulary) to the macro-governmental (see eg Hauck et al, 2003).

Economic principles

One of the assumptions of economics is that of scarcity, which means that we must make choices about how to distribute resources. Resources in this context are not just financial, but also include staff, buildings and infrastructure:

—

> Economics is the study of how humans and society end up choosing, with or without the use of money, to employ scarce productive resources that could have alternative uses, to produce various commodities and distribute them for consumption, now or in the future, among various persons and groups in society. Economics analyses the costs and benefits of improving patterns of resource allocation. (Samuelson, 1980, p 2)

Scarcity of resources means that sacrifices need to be made in the form of alternatives forgone from the consumption of a good or service. This is typically known as the *opportunity cost* of the decision. Opportunity cost is a key concept in health economics and represents the value of the consequences forgone by choosing to deploy a resource in one way rather than in its best alternative use. In its promotion of *efficiency*, health economics can help systems produce more of what they want to produce, for example, increases in population health. In its simplest form, efficiency means providing value for money in the use of resources.

In health economics there are two types of efficiency: *allocative* and *technical*. Allocative efficiency is concerned with how we allocate budgets to achieve the greatest efficiency within a given population or community. Therefore, 'allocative efficiency is achieved when resources are allocated so as to maximise the welfare of the community' (Palmer and Torgerson, 1999, p 1136). Technical efficiency is concerned with how we produce health care services at least cost to the system, whilst achieving maximum health gain. Technical efficiency is achieved 'when the maximum possible improvement in outcome is obtained from a set of resource inputs' (Palmer and Torgerson, 1999, p 1136).

Health economics adopts a normative framework to evaluate the cost-effectiveness of health care services and offers a 'technical' solution to the problem of scarcity of resources by providing decision-makers with recommendations that will help in informing resource allocation decisions.

Economic evaluation

Economic evaluation is one of the major tools used by health economists to explore the cost-effectiveness of interventions. The traditional approach to economic evaluation rests on welfare economics, the fundamental premise being that, where possible, public policy decisions should reflect the preferences of those who will be affected by them. Consequently, the welfare of each individual is the unit of analysis. Economic evaluation allows comparisons of the cost and consequences of different interventions (or service developments) to be made. It explores whether the additional benefits of an intervention are greater than the additional costs (Hauck et al, 2003).

Box 4.1: Key concepts in health economics

Opportunity cost

The value of the consequences forgone by choosing to deploy a resource in one way rather than it best alternative use, that is, it is what you choose not to do that is the opportunity cost.

The goal of resource allocation (within health economics) is to minimise opportunity cost. A recent example is NICE guidance on the use of Bevcizumab (avastin) in the NHS (NICE, 2007). NICE guidance recommended that avastin should not be made available, as while there was some evidence of effect, this was at considerable additional cost and, therefore, the treatment was deemed not to be cost-effective. Thus, resources will not be allocated to fund this drug and the opportunity cost here is the provision of avastin to cancer patients.

Efficiency

Efficiency measures whether health care resources are being used to get the best value for money.

Allocative efficiency refers to allocation of resources across disease areas/patients so as to maximise the level of population health. An example of a question of allocative efficiency is: which conditions should we fund screening for?

Technical efficiency occurs when we produce the maximum possible output for any given set of inputs. Examples of questions of technical efficiency are: what is the most efficient way to screen for breast cancer?

Economic evaluations typically involve making comparisons between two or more options (one option could include doing nothing – ie no treatment). Evaluations must consider both the costs and consequences of interventions. Therefore, cost analysis that takes no account of outcomes is not an economic evaluation in the strict sense. There are four main categories of economic evaluation that are primarily distinguished by their approach to outcomes measurement (for a more detailed discussion, see Gold et al, 1996; Drummond et al, 2005):

- *Cost–benefit analysis (CBA)* measures consequences in monetary terms. CBA is broader in its scope than other approaches, that is, the measure is not restricted to health care as it considers all costs and consequences that affect welfare. Thus, it assigns a cost to both the health and non–health benefits that consumers may derive from health care programmes (Drummond et al, 2005). CBA allows for comparisons across and within programme areas and, as such, can measure both technical and allocative efficiency. This method is not widely used in health care in the UK primarily due to the difficulty in valuing benefits in monetary terms.
- *Cost-effectiveness analysis (CEA)* is traditionally the most commonly used type of economic evaluation. In CEA, costs are measured in monetary terms and

consequences are measured in the most appropriate natural effect or physical unit. Results are reported in terms of cost per unit effect. Examples include: life years saved; life years gained; complications avoided; symptom-free days; and bed days avoided. CEA can address technical efficiency questions and, as such, is limited to a disease or treatment area. For example, in a comparison of the cost-effectiveness of population-based Chlamydia screening compared to targeted or active screening, outcomes were measured in terms of major outcomes avoided (in this case, pelvic inflammation disease) (Roberts et al, 2007). The advantages of CEA are that it is a clear, common and popular technique. Some of the disadvantages of this method are that there are often multiple objectives and no obvious main outcome. Therefore, a choice needs to be made as to which outcome is to be explored in the cost–effectiveness analysis.

- *Cost-minimisation analysis (CMA)* involves the measurement of costs and consequences as in the CEA approach. However, CMA is only adopted if all relevant consequences are deemed to be identical between alternatives so that resources should be allocated to the least costly intervention. An example of a CMA study can be found in the work of Henderson et al (2000). Like CEA, CMA measures outcomes in terms of natural or physical units and, as such, allows us to address issues of technical efficiency.

- *Cost–utility analysis* is a variant of CEA that is characterised by the adoption of summary outcome measures such as Quality-Adjusted Life Years (QALYs) gained. The QALY is a composite measure that combines information on both the length and quality of life. Therefore, the QALY assumes that length and quality of life are both important parameters in health technology assessment. The reasoning underpinning the QALY approach is that, given the choice, a person would be willing to trade off some length of life for a better quality of life. The approach is therefore based on the idea that overall benefit derived from a health intervention or programme can be summarised as the survival benefit weighted to reflect the quality of life in that survival (Williams, 1985). Results are reported in terms of cost per additional QALY gained and can be used to explore both technical and allocative efficiency. The fact that CUA can allow for comparisons to be made across treatment (disease) areas is a major advantage of this approach.

Calculating Quality-Adjusted Life Years

The QALY approach assigns a health-related quality-of-life weight (a value) to each time period. A weight of 1 corresponds to optimal (or perfect) health and 0 is a health state judged to be equivalent to death (Weinstein and Stason, 1977). The QALYs relating to each pathway are expressed as the sum total of the quality weight and time duration. Figure 4.1 provides graphical representation of the two paths. In path A (the 'with treatment' pathway), there is an initial dip in health following treatment, which is followed by health increases until death at eight years. In contrast, Path B (the 'without treatment' pathway) shows a decline in health

Figure 4.1: Quality-Adjusted Life Years gained from an intervention

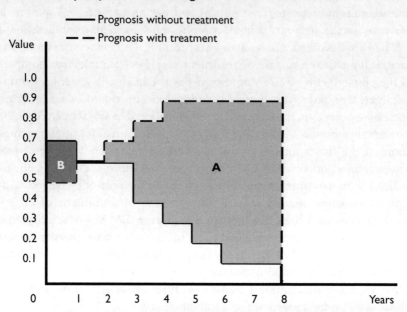

until death at eight years. To assess the impact of the health care intervention the QALYs associated with Path A (6.2) are subtracted from those from Path B (3.0). Thus, the health care intervention produces a QALY gain of 3.2.

In its simplest case the QALY calculation can be represented as:

$$QALY = T_1 Q_1 - T_0 Q_0$$

where T is the number of years of survival and Q_1 and Q_0 represents the health state value with treatment and without treatment, respectively (Tsuchiya and Dolan, 2005).

Two pieces of information are needed to calculate QALYs: the path of the health states over the time span for which the QALYs are to be calculated, and the quality weights that represent the health-related quality of life of the health states that are to be considered. Thus, there are two types of data required to estimate QALYs:

QA = information on health-related quality of life,

LY = information on life years (mortality benefit expressed as life years gained).

Data on life years is relatively easy to obtain from epidemiological sources and life expectancy tables, for example, data on life expectancy at birth by health and local authorities in the United Kingdom can be accessed via the Office for National Statistics. Data on quality of life is more difficult to obtain and there are various instruments that can be used to obtain quality-of-life weights. In essence, these instruments are based on preferences, anchored on perfect health and death, and measured on an interval scale. The four most popular instruments used to measure quality of life include: the Standard Gamble (SG); Time Trade-Off (TTO); Visual Analogue Scale; and the Person Trade-Off (PTO) Technique (for more information on these, see Brazier et al, 1999; Drummond et al, 2005).

Theoretical considerations

It is important that decision-makers are aware of the theoretical framework that underpins the QALY approach as this will influence the decision recommendations produced. The QALY methodology is based on the utilitarian principle outlined in Chapter Two – that is, the imperative to maximise the benefits to society from health care spending – and as such the preferred or recommended course of action is to allocate resources to the intervention that will maximise health gain per pound spent. This efficiency principle sees the interests of the community as more important than the interests of individuals. The theoretical framework of utilitarianism is built on the assumption that individuals are utility-maximisers and that their preferences satisfy the axioms of Expected Utility Theory (EUT). EUT is based on the work of Von Neumann and Morgenstern (1944) and is an approximation to behaviour under uncertainty, which assumes that individuals make choices about different options (in this case health states) in a mathematically predictable and consistent manner, that is, they are logical (McGuire, 2001, p 9).

Put simply, EUT suggests that individuals embody the following five axioms:

1. Completeness of preferences: decision-makers are always able to express a preference when presented with two alternatives.
2. Transitivity of preferences: that is, more is always preferred to less.
3. Monotonicity of preferences: that is, decision-makers will prefer a high probability of outcome above a low probability of outcome.
4. Continuity of preferences: that is, if there were, for example, three choices (1, 2, 3) and the individuals prefers 1 to 2 and 2 to 3 then there must be a possible situation when the decision-maker is indifferent between the mix of 1 and 3 and that a combination of 1 and 3 are equally as good as 2.
5. Substitution of preferences: the assumption that if a decision-maker is indifferent between two outcomes, then they will be indifferent between two lotteries that give them equal outcome probabilities.

EUT is also employed as a conceptual framework for the analysis of decision-making under risk in medicine, finance, economics and insurance (Ecckhoudt, 1996, p 12). It is not intended as a description of how individuals actually make decisions in the face of uncertainty, but as a prescriptive or normative model of how they *ought* to make decisions if they wish to act rationally as defined by the basic axioms (Ecckhoudt, 1996, p 145).

However, there are many criticisms of the utilitarian and EUT approaches to decision-making. Rawls criticises the utilitarian framework for its focus on efficiency and maximising health benefit to the exclusion of distributional factors and the imperative to allocate resources to the worst off (Rawls, 1971). While proponents argue that the QALY approach is 'egalitarian within the health domain; that is, each individual's health is counted equally' (Torrance, 1986, p 17), critics such as Harris (1987) argue that the method favours the young over the old and can discriminate against certain groups in society. As detailed in Chapter Two, the utilitarian approach advocated in these economic methodologies does not take full account of alternative ethical principles such as the rule of rescue.

As well as ethical challenges to the utilitarian approach, the underpinning axioms of EUT have also been challenged – for example, the assertion that individuals act in the rational manner depicted. Furthermore, decision-makers may not have well-constructed preferences that they can easily draw upon when making complex decisions. Box 4.2 outlines some of the main challenges to EUT.

Box 4.2: Challenges to the axioms of expected utility theory

Notion of completeness (axiom 1)
The notion of completeness assumes that individuals are able to articulate and express values for even the most diverse topics. However, other schools of thought suggest that if individuals are faced with an unfamiliar or difficult issue, they are likely to construct preferences rather than draw on informed or existing ones (Fischhoff, 1991). It is important, therefore, to give people time to construct their preferences and consider the implications of these.

Notions of rationality (axioms 2–5)
Axioms 2–5 assume that individuals are able to use available information in a logical and systematic manner in order to maximise utility. Psychologists have challenged this notion and suggest that a number of factors including emotions, attitudes, environment and past experience may all affect the preference-elicitation process. In addition, behaviour may be adaptive and dependent on context (Kahneman and Smith, 2002).

There is also evidence to suggest that individuals struggle to fully analyse complex situations that involve economic and probabilistic judgements, instead relying on heuristics and/or cognitive shortcuts to help them make choices, which could lead to them ignoring relevant and important information (Payne et al, 1992). This bounded rationality increases with the complexity of the task (Simon, 1978).

Limitations in the theoretical underpinnings of the QALY need to be considered by those who are intending to use this approach to inform decisions, and the danger is that uncritical adoption becomes engrained in priority-setting decisions. For example, the utilitarian pursuit of health maximisation may not be compatible with the broader values informing decision–making. QALY calculations can be modified to incorporate other instrumental values (eg relating to age and lifestyle), but only if those conducting the analysis are competent in the analytical techniques involved in weighting QALYs (Wagstaff, 1991; Williams, 1997).

Methodological considerations

This section considers three areas of tension relating to the methodologies of economic evaluation. These are:

- Whose values should be incorporated into the QALY calculation?
- Which health state valuation techniques should be used?
- How should evidence be elicited?

Whose values?

There is much debate in the literature around whose values (ie patients, general public or experts) are most appropriate to inform cost-per-QALY calculations. There are three ways to obtain quality-of-life data to inform QALYs, these include:

- *Using expert opinion to estimate quality-of-life values.* This is a relatively cheap and easy way to obtain data. However, this data is likely to be subjective and prone to bias. Further, if the interest is in being accountable to the population, then public values may be more appropriate (Dolan, 2000).
- *Using published quality-of-life values.* This could involve reviewing studies that have recorded values for the disease or intervention of interest. If this approach is adopted, then it is important that the health states used in the study match the ones of interest. Similarly, subjects sampled in previous studies need to be similar and comparable to the subjects of interest (ie elderly people and teenagers may view health states differently). Further, it is important to check that the measurement instruments used in studies are credible. The University of York conducted a population-based exercise that used the time trade-off technique to collect population-based values for health states in England. These are a readily available resource that can be used to estimate the quality-of-life aspects of QALYs (Dolan et al, 1995). The York population valuations have been applied to a number of published studies and are used to inform economic evaluations conducted by NICE.
- *Obtaining patient quality-of-life values.* This is time-consuming and costly and it may not always be possible or appropriate. Studies have also shown that patients may well value health states differently than the general population (Dolan, 2000).

The decision around 'Whose values?' may rest on the decision-making arena. For example, if making comparisons of interventions for the same condition, then it may be appropriate to use patient values, but if making decisions about comparisons across different diseases and sub-populations, then it may be more appropriate to use general population valuations. In a publically funded system such as the NHS, it is often suggested that the preferences of those who pay for health care (ie the public) should be used to inform resource allocation decisions (Broome, 1991; Dolan, 2000). The Washington expert panel on economic evaluation techniques recommends:

> Reference case analyses from the societal perspective for purposes of resource allocation should use the health state preferences of a well-informed, cognitively robust, unbiased community sample. Although pristine weights are currently available, preferences from a community sample are, on balance the most appropriate source. (Gold et al, 1996, p 106)

Which health state valuation technique?

A further contentious area concerns which method is most appropriate for eliciting the values individuals attach to different health states. Studies have shown that using different techniques such as the Standard Gamble (SG), Time Trade-off (TTO), Visual Analogue Scale (VAS) and Person Trade-Off Technique (PTO) can produce very different results and thus potentially impact on the overall resource allocation decision. The literature around the methodological and empirical issues relating to the different techniques is vast, with mixed views on which technique should be used in QALY calculations. Some commentators suggest that the SG technique is the most appropriate as it incorporates notions of risk and uncertainty – and, as such, is based on the fundamental axioms of utility theory that underpin the QALY approach. The TTO approach was developed by Torrance (1971) to overcome some of the practical difficulties of probabilities associated with the SG method. However, the fact that this approach does not include notions of risk and uncertainty leads some to suggest that it is an inferior method to the SG approach and is not consistent with expected utility theory (for further discussion, see Torrance, 1971). Data on validity and reliability of techniques suggest that SG and TTO are the most valid and reliable measures. Further details on the accuracy and validity of techniques can be found in Brazier et al (1999), Nord (1991) and Robinson (1999).

The elicitation process

A further area of methodological interest relates to the process of eliciting health state valuations as there is some suggestion that the mode of delivery may affect the overall health state valuation. Methods include self-completion and interviewer-administered questionnaires, which can be conducted with or without deliberation (either individual or collective). If, as Fischoff (1991) suggests, individuals do not have well-informed preferences to call upon when valuing health states, the use of deliberative processes can be important in enabling individuals to reflect on and construct their preferences during the elicitation process. Thus, the process of administration may actually aid the construction of preferences as well as elicit them, and discrepancies in results may therefore be a function of a deliberative process of reflection rather than measurement error (Shiell et al, 2000).

The Disability-Adjusted Life Year

The Disability-Adjusted Life Year (DALY) measure, which was first introduced in the late 1990s by the World Bank, combines the number of years lost due to premature death (years of life lost – YLL) and the number of years lived with a disability (YLD). DALYs have two purposes:

- to calculate the global burden of disease – this is a positive exercise (ie how things are); and
- to be used as an outcome measure in cost-effective analysis – this is a normative exercise (ie includes value judgements).

DALYs use disability weights to reflect the burden associated with living in particular health states. In the DALY approach, each state of health is assigned a disability weighting on a scale from 0 (perfect health) to 1 (death). The disability weight is a utility weight similar to that of the health state utility weight used in the QALY. However, the scales are opposite to the health state utility weight used

Figure 4.2: QALYs and DALYs

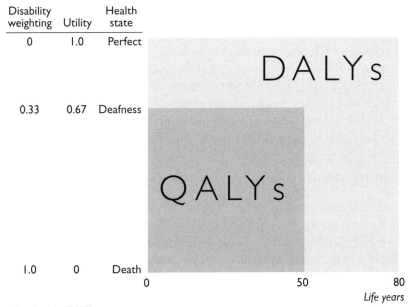

Source: Fox-Rushby (2002)

to calculate QALYs. Thus, one wants less DALYs and more QALYs: by definition DALYs are a 'bad' that should be minimised (Anand and Hanson, 1997).

Conceptually, QALYs and DALYs are very similar in that both are composite health outcome measures combining quality and duration of life, and many of the often-mentioned differences between them are not essential differences. For example, criticisms of the valuation method – the use of experts as subjects to perform the valuation task – the discounting and the age weights, as operationalised in the Global Burden of Disease (GBD) study are not essential to the concept (Murray et al, 2000). They refer to choices in the derivation process of DALYs and were choices made in the GBD study (World Health Organization, 2000; for further discussion of the DALY used in the GBD study, see also Fox-Rushby, 2002; Essink-Bot et al, 2002).

Williams (1999) notes that the distinction between QALYs and DALYs is often blurred and he describes DALYs as a 'variant' of the QALY approach. One of the main differences between the QALY and the DALY is the way health is conceptualised. DALYs focus on disease and use a disease-specific description of health, whereas QALYs tend to use a generic health description that focuses on various dimensions of health. This focus on disease means that DALYs are less inclusive than QALYs. For example, DALYs do not include side effects, co-morbidities or the ability to adapt to conditions before and after treatment, all of which can be captured in a QALY (Fox-Rushby, 2002).

Information on prevalence and incidence of disease is required in the calculation of DALYs, which therefore require high-quality epidemiological data to formulate burden-of-disease estimates. This information is then imputed into the disease pathway model (Kruijshar et al, 2004). However, epidemiological data is often unavailable and varies between countries and even within regions of a country (Essink-Bot et al, 2002; Kruijshar et al, 2004). The majority of studies that have used DALYs in economic evaluations tend to be from developing countries and often have limited relevance outside of these settings. Furthermore, unlike QALYs, there are no published population valuations. Perhaps for these reasons, DALYs have not had the 'success' of QALYs in terms of uptake. Further, they require more effort in that they need to incorporate epidemiological information on the prevalence and incidence of a disease. Thus, the time and effort needed to calculate DALYs may not in itself be cost-effective (Williams, 1999).

Presenting results

Full economic evaluations (ie CEA, CMA, CUA and CBA) take an incremental approach to measuring the costs and effects of an intervention/technology. As such an incremental economic evaluation answers the following question: 'What is the difference in costs and the difference in consequences of option A compared to option B?'

Thus, the interest is in the additional cost per unit of outcome achieved when comparing one treatment to another. This is called the Incremental Cost-

Effectiveness Ratio (ICER), which simply involves calculating the difference in cost by the difference in outcome (see Box 4.3).

Box 4.3: The Incremental Cost-Effectiveness Ratio

The ICER is calculated as follows:

$$ICER = \frac{\text{Difference in costs}}{\text{Difference in consequences}}$$

For example:

$$ICER = \frac{£40,000 - £20,000}{5 - 3 \text{ 'units' gained}} = £10,000 \text{ per 'unit'}$$

This calculation is then plotted on to the incremental cost-effectiveness plane, as shown in the following figure:

Figure 4.3: The cost-effectiveness plane

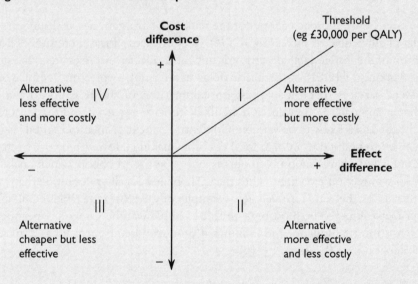

If the ICER calculation ends up in quadrant II or IV, then the choices are relatively clear. In quadrant II the new intervention is more effective and less costly and, as such, dominates the alternative, so the decision would be that it is cost-effective. If the intervention is in quadrant IV, then the opposite is true. In quadrants I and III, the choice depends on the maximum cost-effectiveness ratio a decision-maker is willing to accept (eg £30,000 per QALY).

The results from economic evaluations are generally used in two ways: threshold approaches and league tables.

The threshold approach

The threshold approach involves comparing the ICER to a critical threshold value. This approach is used by NICE, who have a cost per QALY threshold of around £20,000–£30,000 (NICE, 2010). One of the weaknesses of this approach is that it does not consider the notion of affordability. This, it is argued, could lead to increased spending and inefficient allocation of resources (Gafni and Birch, 2006). Technologies may well have favourable ICERs and yet may not be considered affordable to the health care system, and recommendations may well ignore the opportunity cost to a health economy (Klein, 2010). In practice, decision-makers faced with favourable ICERs may therefore need to undertake further budgetary impact analysis (Cohen, 2006). There are also concerns that the objectives of decision-makers may be at odds with the ICER calculation, with the latter being an insufficient basis for decision-making in health care, and that their use, therefore, may actually fail to maximise health gains within a given budget constraint (Birch and Gafni, 2006; Cohen, 2006).

QALY league tables

The cost–utility approach allows for the ranking of programmes/technologies in order of efficiency (or increasing ICER). This involves allocating resources from the top of the league table downwards until all available resources are exhausted. The ranking of ICERs is problematic as it does not involve any comparison between services to be made, just the comparison of the ICER. In practice, different approaches to evaluation are likely to have occurred and the level and quality of data is likely to be variable. Context-specific data are important if league tables are to be used to inform local decision-making. However, priority setters are unlikely to have the time, resources and expertise to conduct such analyses, and so will rely on existing studies that may be less locally relevant. Perhaps for these reasons, there are relatively few examples of QALY league tables being used in priority setting. The most high-profile example was the Oregon experiment, which is most famous for the rankings it produced being received as clinically counter-intuitive (Hadorn, 1991b).

Resources for priority setters

Not all priority setters can be expected to have the skills or resources to conduct their own formal economic evaluations and they will therefore be reliant on externally commissioned or 'off-the-shelf' analyses. There are a number of existing health and social care resources that provide information on different types of economic data. For example, the websites of NICE and the Health Technology Assessment programme provide details of economic evaluations. Other sites such as the Health Economics Evaluations Database (HEED) contain details of both nationally and internationally published studies. For those who wish to

—

conduct local studies, the Personal Social Services Research Unit (PSSRU) and NHS reference costs provide national cost data that can be used in economic evaluation – this can be used when local data is inaccurate or missing and/or when comparisons between local and national data need to be made. Table 4.1 provides further details on organisations that provide economic information.

Table 4.1: UK organisations that provide economic information

Organisation	Outline of available resource	Website
National Institute of Health and Clinical Excellence (NICE)	Provides guidance on the clinical and cost-effectiveness of new and existing medicines, treatments and procedures in the NHS.	www.nice.org.uk/
Social Care Institute for Excellence (SCIE), an independent charity funded by the Department of Health and the devolved administrations in Wales and Northern Ireland	Identifies and disseminates the knowledge base for good practice in social care. Although SCIE does not conduct economic evaluations it does identify resources.	www.scie.org.uk/
Health Technology Assessment (HTA) Programme	The HTA programme produces independent research about the effectiveness of different health care treatments and tests for those who use, manage and provide care in the NHS.	www.hta.ac.uk/
Health Economic Evaluations Database (HEED)	Contains extensive information on national and international studies that have conducted economic evaluations of treatments and medical interventions.	http://onlinelibrary.wiley.com/book/10.1002/9780470510933
The Centre for Reviews and Dissemination (CRD) (based at the University of York and part of the National Institute for Health Research)	Undertakes systematic reviews that evaluate the effects of health and social care interventions. It is also home to the following databases – *DARE, NHS EED and HTA* – which provide details on economic reviews and Health Technology Assessments.	www.york.ac.uk/inst/crd/
Health information resources (formerly the National Library for Health)	Provides extensive access to studies conducted in health and social care.	www.library.nhs.uk/Default.aspx
NHS reference costs	NHS reference costs are published yearly and provide information on NHS expenditure, including unit costs, average length of stay and activity levels.	www.dh.gov.uk
Personal Social Services Research Unit (PSSRU)	Provides data on the unit costs of health and social care that can be used in economic evaluations.	www.pssru.ac.uk

For those seeking to critique or evaluate the quality of economic evaluations there are a number of helpful checklists, which are outlined in Table 4.2.

Table 4.2: Economic evaluation checklists for published studies

British Medical Journal (BMJ)	Authors guide to submission of economic evaluations. Contains a series of questions around what is expected of a high-quality economic evaluation. Available at: http://resources.bmj.com/bmj/authors/checklists-forms/health-economics
Drummond et al (2005)	Similar to the BMJ checklist, this resource provides a series of questions that relate to economic evaluation methodology and help reviewers to critique studies.
Critical Appraisal Skills Programme (CASP)	This tool adapts the Drummond et al (2005) checklist and provides a series of questions that explore the validity and reliability of economic evaluations as well as the generalisability of results to local settings. Available at: http://www.casp-birmingham.org/

Using economic evaluation in priority setting

Economic evaluations feature highly in the outputs of national guidance-producing agencies such as NICE. However, this picture is typically not replicated amongst those actually allocating budgets. For example, a number of studies have been conducted into the actual impact of economic evaluation on technology coverage decisions at local levels of health care (Eddama and Coast, 2009). These reveal low levels of usage to a remarkable degree of consistency across international contexts and over time. This is despite most studies reporting receptiveness to greater usage among respondents, and outlining numerous strategies for improved access and expertise among decision-makers. A major issue for local decision-makers is the time and cost involved in actually undertaking good-quality economic evaluations. Analysis can involve very complex and sophisticated modelling techniques that require specialist inputs. The complexity involved in modelling in economic analysis and some of the uncertainty and assumptions around the data inputs can be a barrier to the use of economic analysis. As well as access and expertise deficits, research suggests that decision-makers are often sceptical of analyses that are produced by manufacturers of technologies.

In a study of local decision-making committees in the NHS, Williams and Bryan (2007a) found that only a small percentage of local technology coverage committees routinely requested economic evaluations and that accessing analyses was an even less frequent occurrence. At local levels, there was little or no health economics expertise available to interpret evaluations, or apparent inclination to act on their recommendations. As well as confirming the barriers mentioned earlier, this study uncovered other aspects of decision-making contexts that appeared to inhibit the use of economic evaluation. The first area of uncertainty concerned the criteria by which decisions were made. It was not clear, for example, on whose behalf decisions were made and therefore to whom decision-makers were accountable. The second area of uncertainty related to institutional and financial responsibilities. For example, in each case it was not clear whether or how implementation of decisions taken would be resourced. Similarly, the extent to which decisions made were adhered to by clinicians seemed to depend more on exhortation than compulsion, and there was no formal requirement of the organisations involved to adopt the recommendations produced by the priority-setting exercise. A third area of potential confusion related to the processes followed by committees. For example, it was not clear how evidence would be gathered and fed into decisions, how interest groups would be engaged or how decisions would be disseminated and reviewed. In this context, it is difficult to know at what stage economic considerations would or should be brought to bear on deliberations. These findings suggest that the decision-making context needs to be compatible with economic evaluations if the latter are to be useful.

Economic evaluations follow an evidence-based model of priority setting that conforms to the rationalist model outlined in Chapter One. In particular, these can be understood in the context of the broader evidence-based movement in health care that 'draws on "science" and all its modernist trappings of truth and progress and is presented as rational and politically neutral' (Harrison, 1998, p 21).

While it is difficult to argue against evidence-based decision-making, as we have seen, this comes with caveats. Box 4.4 provides a checklist of questions that may be helpful for decision-makers who need to decide which evidence is relevant to their priority-setting task.

Box 4.4: The evidence-based model of priority setting

Building on the work of Glasby et al (2007a), we propose the following checklist of questions for decision-makers who need to decide which evidence is relevant to their priority-setting task:

- What constitutes valid evidence?
- Is the evidence from a reliable source?
- Are certain types of evidence to be treated as more legitimate than others?
- What happens when evidence is fragmented or contradictory?
- Is the available evidence relevant to the decision?
- Is the available evidence relevant to the local setting?
- How much evidence does there need to be before we can be confident about a particular prioritisation decision?

Lomas et al (2005, p 9) note that 'evidence is inherently uncertain, dynamic, complex, contestable and rarely complete'. Therefore, if it is to be used in priority setting, then some form of deliberation that tests the merits and limitations of the evidence and its usefulness and impact on the decision in question is needed. Explicit deliberation involves making the validation and critique of information more transparent and open to other stakeholder considerations.

As well as helping to inform decisions, the appeal to best evidence can also help to persuade stakeholders – such as clinicians and managers – of both the validity and importance of priority setting through its emphasis on rigorous medical research, which uses quantitative analyses such as systematic reviews and randomised controlled trials (RCTs) (Jenkings and Barber, 2004). However, while such quantitative evidence is important to priority setting – that is, in providing important information on the incidence and prevalence of a disease and/or the cost of interventions – the use of other types of research as well as tacit knowledge or practice can also have an important role to play (Kovner et al, 2000). For example, if the interest is in patients' views around satisfaction and quality of services, then an RCT or systematic review is most likely to have not considered such views and is therefore not fit for this purpose.

Glasby et al (2007a) challenge the traditional hierarchy of evidence framework and call for a broader notion of *'knowledge-based practice'* that includes both quantitative and qualitative research as well as the experiential expertise of practitioners and service users.

Economic evaluation and social care

While there has been an increase in the number of economic evaluations in health care, there is an imbalance between evaluations for health interventions and those for social care (Knapp, 1999; McDaid et al, 2003). The lack of economic evidence in social care is due in part to the complex nature of social welfare interventions, including: 'a high degree of user involvement, significant variability within the programme, complex long term conditions and multiagency involvement' (McDaid et al, 2003, p 96). A recent review on social care for older people in England developed a new measure called the Activities of Daily Living Adjusted Year (ADLAY), which attempts to incorporate measures of daily living that the QALY may be unable to capture (Wanless, 2006, p xxvii). The authors suggest that the criteria used to inform the cost-effectiveness analysis is 'an approach which mirrors that used by the NICE for new health care interventions' (Humphries et al, 2010, p 43). There are currently few published studies that have used this approach and an absence of published critique.

Another measure that has been developed by the PSSRU for use in the social care arena is the Adult Social Care Outcomes Toolkit (ASCOT) (PSSRU, 2010). ASCOT is intended to capture information on the individual's social care-related quality of life (SCRQOL). The development of the measure is in response to the lack of sensitivity of current measures, such as QALYs, to aspects of SCRQOL (Netton et al, 2010). There are four measures used in the ASCOT that should be applied according to individual circumstances and settings (see Box 4.5 for further details). The tool can be used to assess the cost-effectiveness of social care interventions and services.

Box 4.5: The four versions of the ASCOT

SCT4: The four-level self-completion tool is for use with people who live in community settings. It has nine four-level questions from which current SCRQOL can be calculated.

INT4: The four-level interview tool is for use with people who live in community settings. It has 23 questions from which current SCRQOL and expected SCRQOL can be calculated.

SCT3: The three-level self-completion tool is for use with people who live in community settings. It has 18 questions that calculate current SCRQOL and can generate predicted SCRQOL gain from indirect indicators based on previous research in a day care setting. These indicators have not been tested for appropriateness outside of the day care setting.

CH3: The toolkit is for use in residential settings. Using a combination of observation (CHOBS3) and interviews with residents, relatives and staff (CHINT3), both current and expected SCRQOL can be calculated.

Source: Netton et al (2010).

The developers of this toolkit have carried out validation tests that show positive results, but further independent studies and applications are required (Caiels et al, 2010). Further access to the ASCOT tool can be obtained via the PSSRU website.

Learning exercise 4.1: Economic evaluation self-test

Which economic evaluation technique/s allow for comparisons of:

- technical efficiency?
- allocative efficiency?

What benefits do economic techniques such as cost-effectiveness and cost–utility analysis have to offer resource allocation in health care?

What are some of the weaknesses associated with economic evaluation as an aid to resource allocation in health care?

What are the strengths and weaknesses of the QALY measure as a tool for priority setting?

Chapter summary

Economic evaluation (as part of health technology assessment) has long been advocated as a tool to support priority setting in health care and it is particularly suited to decisions regarding technology coverage. However, decision-makers should be aware of the principles underpinning economic evaluation and how these have been challenged, as well as the limitations of the methods used to elicit values and construct outcome measures. It is also important to acknowledge the resource-intensive nature of economic evaluation and decision-makers should consider issues of scale and scope when allocating resources to the generation and/or accessing of formal cost-effectiveness analyses. As with other decision inputs discussed in previous chapters, there is also a need to consider how the role of formal analyses is incorporated into an overall decision process. The relatively low rate of actual usage of economic evaluation at local levels is a cause for concern. A range of barriers prevent the full use of these techniques and these include shortages in analytical skills and infrastructure, as well as weaknesses in the methods themselves. However, despite these limitations, sufficient evidence exists of a desire on the part of decision-makers for decision analysis to support the priority-setting process (see eg Mitton and Donaldson, 2001; Robinson et al, 2011b). The following chapter introduces a series of tools designed to better reflect the realities of the decision-making environment in which priority setters are located and that allow stakeholders to develop multiple assessment criteria with which to assess new and existing health care interventions.

FIVE

Multi-criteria decision analysis and priority-setting processes

Key points covered in Chapter Five

- Multi-criteria decision analysis (MCDA) is increasingly used as part of health care priority setting. This approach typically combines a wider range of considerations than is included within mainstream economic evaluation.
- MCDA approaches range from relatively simple scorecard tools to more sophisticated computer-based modelling.
- Multi-criteria approaches can also be used in processes such as programme budgeting and marginal analysis. Typically, such processes involve input from decision stakeholders and are based on economic principles such as opportunity cost and marginal analysis.
- These approaches are useful, but are not sufficient for successful priority setting. Limitations include: data shortages; difficulties in incentivising participation; and problems of the subsequent implementation of decisions.

Introduction

In this chapter, we introduce tools and examples that attempt to combine a broader range of the considerations involved in priority setting than is typically facilitated by economic evaluation. These include: multi-criteria approaches (such as the Portsmouth scorecard and the socio-technical approach), programme budgeting and marginal analysis (PBMA), and ethical frameworks, all of which have been used by commissioning organisations in the English NHS. Broadly speaking, these approaches sacrifice some of the *rigour* associated with the discipline of health economics in order to maximise *relevance* to the decision-making context. This chapter also signposts resources available to NHS priority setters seeking to draw on these different approaches.

Multi-criteria approaches

Multi-criteria decision approaches are increasingly used as part of formal decision-making processes in a number of sectors including health care (Hirschberg et al, 2004; Baltussen et al, 2006; Mendoza and Martins, 2006). These typically allow for consideration and analysis of multiple streams of often very different information, including economic and financial data as well as other relevant factors such as the number intended to be treated and equity. Belton and Stewart (2002, p 2) define MCDA as 'an umbrella term to describe a collection of formal approaches which seek to take explicit account of multiple criteria in helping individuals or groups explore decisions that matter'.

The main function of MCDA is to help decision-makers to organise and synthesise a variety of information relevant to the decision-making question. It is therefore intended to aid the decision-making process by integrating objective measurement with value judgements, and, in the process, making explicit the value positions held by decision-makers. In this way, the often implicit ethical injunctions informing priority setting can be explicitly considered. However, it is not intended to replace deliberation and judgement. Belton and Stewart (2002, p 3) note that MCDA is not able to 'provide the "right" answer to the decision question, provide an "objective" analysis that moves the responsibility of the decision maker or take the pain out of making difficult decisions'.

The process of MCDA, as outlined by Belton and Stewart (2002), has three distinct phases: problem structuring; model building; and informing and challenging thinking:

- *Problem structuring:* this phase attempts to identify the problems and issues that are relevant to the priority-setting decision in question. It can be used to identify a number of relevant aspects, such as: important services areas; current patient pathways; interventions suitable for evaluation; strategic aims of health care organisations; and alignment of these with other stakeholder perspectives. It is also the stage at which the values and goals of individuals, organisations and stakeholder groups are identified. For this phase, important things to consider include: which stakeholders should be involved in the process; and what types of events will be most appropriate.
- *Model building:* this phase focuses on reaching agreement as to the criteria that should be included in the decision model, building on outcomes of the problem structuring phase. These discussions should inform the development of the relevant criteria and subsequent weights applied. Peacock et al (2009) suggest that when agreeing the criteria by which alternatives should be valued, the important questions are: what priority-setting objectives do decision-makers wish to pursue? And what relevant local decision-making criteria should be used to judge decisions? Priority-setting decisions often involve a wide and diverse range of criteria, and decision-makers are required to make trade-offs between these (Peacock et al, 2009). Clearly, in order to avoid double counting, the criteria need to be mutually independent.
- *Challenging thinking:* finally, phase three involves using the model to inform and challenge thinking around decision-making in general as well as specific decisions. This can involve exploration of the validity, robustness and sensitivity of the weights (values) applied on the resource allocation decision.

Within these distinct phases, there are a number of different activities taking place, and the complexity and sophistication of MCDA models vary considerably. The simple linear evaluation model multiplies the values for each criterion by the weight of that criterion and then adds all the weighted scores together. More complex models incorporate a pairwise comparison of the different criteria for each of the different options. For example, a decision-maker will be asked how important one criterion is to another in relation to each of the decisions being made (Baltussen et al, 2006).

Figure 5.1: Stages of MCDA

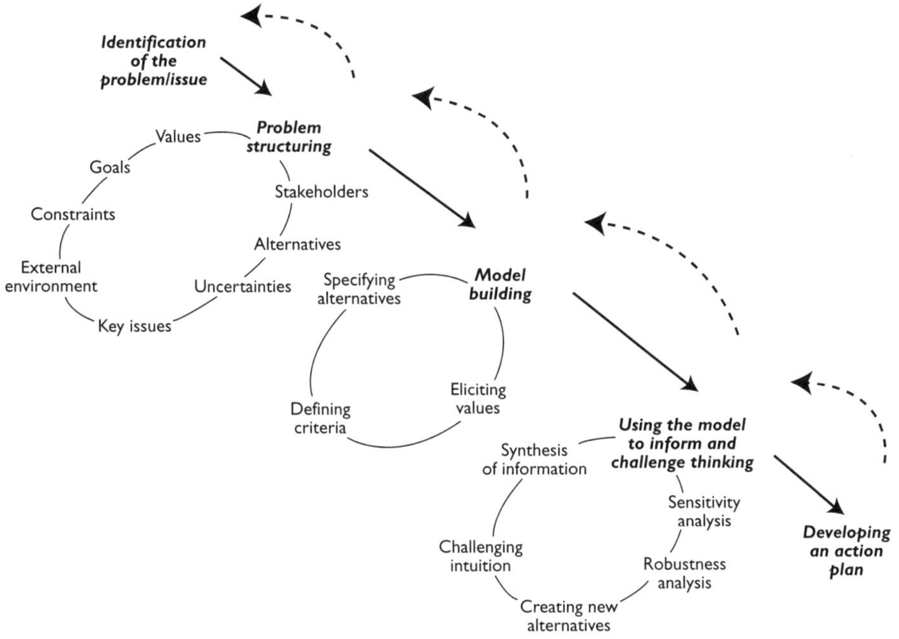

Source: Belton and Stewart (2002)

There are many different MCDA techniques (see Stewart, 1992; Lootsma, 1999; Mendoza and Martins, 2006). In health care these include: the Portsmouth and modified Portsmouth scorecard techniques, and the socio-technical approach. One of the strengths of MCDA is that it allows for the inclusion of a variety of relevant stakeholders to form part of the decision-making body that informs the eventual allocation of health care resources. However, while the MCDA approach has gained in popularity over recent years, there are a number of limitations in relation to its application in priority setting and resource allocation. Many of the criticisms echo those levied at other evidence-based approaches – for example, there is often a lack of valid, reliable and robust local data to populate models, and the development of models can be time and resource intensive. Before a decision can be reached, individuals and organisations need to provide evidence and data in relation to investment and disinvestment decisions for each of the agreed criteria, then experts need to attend panel sessions to score the criteria. These activities require significant time and resources from those involved. The following sections introduce a selection of MCDA approaches in more detail.

The Portsmouth scorecard

The Portsmouth scorecard is a simple tool in so far as it does not tend to involve any sophisticated quantitative analysis. The original Portsmouth scorecard was used to inform decisions around clinical treatments and procedures, and modified versions have since been developed to inform decisions over both clinical and non-clinical interventions in a number of localities across England (Robinson et al, 2011b). As with PBMA, the Portsmouth scorecard has tended to be applied to decisions regarding the funding of new service developments rather than for decisions around core spend or disinvestment. Different versions of the Portsmouth scorecard contain different criteria and apply different weights to these. However, typically these scorecards are designed to assess requests for investment by collecting information on:

* clinical and cost-effectiveness;
* numbers of patients who would benefit;
* clinical engagement in the proposal for investment; and
* risks of not funding the intervention.

Each question has a maximum score and thresholds for scoring within each category. For example, higher scores are often attributed to submissions that demonstrate good-quality clinical evidence from randomised controlled trials (RCTs). Scoring usually involves calculating a single index score for each intervention and then ranking interventions accordingly. Interventions are then placed in rank order whereby the highest-scoring interventions take priority. In theory, this league table of interventions should be funded from first to last until all available resources are utilised.

The appeal of this approach is that it is relatively easy to understand and the criteria can be adapted to suit the local priority-setting context. There is also evidence to suggest that the tool can be used as a vehicle to engage different stakeholder groups in the priority-setting process (Robinson et al, 2009). However, there have been a number of criticisms of this approach. First, there is the familiar issue of evidence deficits. Even when published evidence is available to populate the tool, it is not always applicable to the local setting. Current applications of the Portsmouth scorecard have not tended to test the sensitivity of results (Robinson et al, 2009). Studies also suggest that priority setters have at times expected the Portsmouth scorecard to take the subjectivity out of the decision-making process (Robinson et al, 2011b). However, in practice MCDA techniques are intended to facilitate, rather than replace, decision-making (Belton and Stewart, 2002).

Table 5.1: An example of a modified Portsmouth scorecard

Factor	Very low	Mid-scale	Very high	Score	Maximum points
Magnitude of benefit (health gain)	Under 3 points Limited improvement in health or life expectancy	20 points Moderate improvement in health or life expectancy	40 points Large improvement in health or life expectancy		40
Addresses health inequality	Under 3 points Does not address a health inequality	20 points Partially addresses a health inequality	40 points Fully addresses a health inequality		40
Strength of evidence of clinical effectiveness	Under 3 points Limited or no evidence (case series, experimental)	20 points Modest evidence (cohort studies)	40 points Good evidence (meta-analysis, RCTs)		40
Cost-effectiveness	Under 3 points >£20,000 per QALY	20 points £10–20,000 per QALY	40 points <£10,000 per QALY		40
Number who will benefit	Under 3 points 10	20 points 1,000	40 points 10,000		40
Affordability	Under 3 points >£100,000	10 points <£50,000	20 points Cost saving to the PCT		40
Total					240

Source: Adapted from Southwark PCT (2009, pp 13–14).

Decision conferencing

An example of a priority-setting tool that incorporates MCDA is the socio-technical approach (STA) recently developed by the London School of Economics and piloted in the English NHS (The Health Foundation, 2010). The STA is designed to incorporate technical and social aspects into the decision-making process. The technical dimension is informed by medical, economic and epidemiological evidence, while the social dimension encourages discussion and interpretation of evidence in the light of professional and organisational values.

The STA approach recognises the need to engage stakeholders from across the health economy (including patients, clinicians, local authorities, the voluntary sector, commissioners, nurses and GPs). The process typically involves two one-day stakeholders' events organised as decision conferences. The aim of such events is 'for the stakeholders to declare where investment is needed and how best to deploy it' (The Health Foundation, 2010, p 3). The intention here is for the problem and potential solution to be 'owned' by the stakeholders rather than having been imposed on them by outside agencies.

In the NHS case study sites, stakeholder workshops included representatives from across the health economy, with separate events being held for different disease areas. In the first of the two events, stakeholders identified options to be assessed (current and/or new interventions). Stage two involved a priority-setting event in which these interventions were reviewed by a stakeholder panel. MCDA was then employed using decision conferencing techniques to build decision models. This involved more sophisticated mathematical modelling of quantitative data than is typically used by other MCDA approaches such as the Portsmouth scorecard. Electronic decision conferencing using real-time computer modelling enabled results from a decision model to be displayed and modified continuously during the workshops. Modification involves inputting existing appropriate data into the various criteria (eg data on finance, cost-effectiveness and prevalence of disease) and drawing on expert knowledge from participants to populate the model when relevant information is not available. Decision-makers are required to judge and score each of the different criteria using a previously determined scoring system or include blanks if they do not feel qualified (see Bots and Hulshof, 2000). Individual scores can then be averaged and a group score shown on the conferencing screen. Decision conferencing has been applied for over three decades in different industries and participants highlight that:

> (1) they helped the group to generate a shared understanding of the issues, without requiring consensus about all the issues, (2) they developed a sense of common purpose, while allowing individual differences in perspective, and (3) they gained commitment to the way forward, yet preserving individual paths. (Phillips, 2007, pp 380–1)

Other projects that have used similar methods to inform priority setting in health care have found the process to be both feasible to implement and supported by stakeholders (Dennis et al, 1988; Nunamaker et al, 1997). The STA applied at the NHS pilot sites used the data generated at stage two to estimate Value for Money (VFM) scores – VFM scores are calculated for each pound spent on an intervention. Benefit calculations include information on: length and quality of life, the number of people to benefit, and contribution to reducing inequalities. VFM scores can also be determined along a pathway of care and may help explain differences in relative VFM scores. On the basis of the analysis, one Primary Care Trust reallocated £1m of additional resources and another designed a new strategy to shift investments from residential care to community care for patients with eating disorders. However, results also suggest that the application of such techniques does not necessarily lead to the implementation of proposed changes to service delivery. This stage requires other strategies, as outlined in the following chapter.

Programme budgeting and marginal analysis

PBMA is a formal process for setting priorities and allocating resources that has become increasingly prevalent in health care in the UK and internationally

(Bate and Mitton, 2006). In recent years, the Department of Health in England has advocated its use in commissioning more generally (Department of Health, 2009). PBMA draws on the two economic principles of opportunity cost and marginal analysis. The primary concern is with assessing costs and benefits at the margins, and the focus is on the 'benefit gained from the next unit of resources or lost from having one unit less' (Donaldson et al, 2010, p 2). PBMA attempts to overcome some of the barriers associated with the use of economic evaluations by adopting more flexible, accessible and locally appropriate techniques to inform decision analysis. For example, PBMA is able to accommodate non–utilitarian considerations that may be relevant to priority setting (Klein, 2010) and places a strong emphasis on the involvement of relevant stakeholder groups in the decision-making process.

There are a number of different PBMA formats, but the framework generally asks the following five questions around resource usage (Donaldson et al, 2010, p 4):

1. What resources are available in total?
2. In what ways are these resources currently being spent?
3. What are the main candidates for more resources and what would be their effectiveness and cost?
4. Are there any areas of care within the programme that could be provided to the same level of effectiveness but with less resources, thereby releasing those resources to fund candidates resulting from question 3 (technical efficiency)?
5. Are there areas of care that, despite being effective, should have less resources because a proposal (or proposals) from question 3 is (are) more effective for the resources spent (allocative efficiency)?

A PBMA study consists of seven stages that involve the use of specific programme budgeting techniques to construct a map of current activity and expenditure (outlined in Box 5.1).

Box 5.1: The seven stages of PBMA

1. *Determine the aim and scope of the priority-setting exercise.* This stage determines whether PBMA will be used to examine changes in services within a given programme (micro-/within-programme study design) or between programmes (macro-/between-programme study design).

2. *Compile a programme budget.* In this stage, resources and costs of programmes are identified and quantified. When combined with activity information, these make up the programme budget.

3. *Form a marginal analysis advisory panel.* In this stage, a panel of 8–30 people, made up of key stakeholders, is formed to advise the priority-setting process.

4. *Determine locally relevant decision-making criteria.* In this stage, criteria (eg maximising benefits, improving access and equity, reducing waiting times etc) are elicited from the advisory panel, with reference to national, regional and local objectives, and specified objectives of the local health economy.

5. *Identify options for (a) service growth, (b) resource release from gains in operational efficiencies and (c) resource release from scaling back or ceasing some services.* In this stage, the programme budget, along with information on decision-making objectives, evidence on benefits from service, changes in local health care needs and policy guidance, are used to highlight options for investment and disinvestment.

6. *Evaluate investments and disinvestments.* This stage involves evaluation in terms of costs and benefits and the making of recommendations for (a) funding growth areas with new resources and (b) moving resources from 5(b) and 5(c) to 5(a).

7. *Validate results and reallocate resources.* In this stage, those involved re-examine and validate evidence and judgements used in the process and reallocate resources according to cost–benefit ratios and other decision-making criteria.

Source: Peacock et al (2009 p 125).

There are two measurement phases in the PBMA approach. One involves programme budgeting and the other marginal analysis.

Programme budgeting

The aim behind programme budgeting is to provide a map of how resources are currently being spent. It enables commissioners to see data on whole spend and spend in relation to different practices. This enables comparison between localities of levels of spending on, for example, treatment for heart disease. It also allows for discussions around variations in patterns of expenditure. In order to conduct programme budgeting, data on expenditure and outcomes is required. In England, such data is currently available via the Department of Health who have developed 23 programme budget areas (see Table 5.2).

—

Table 5.2: Programme budget categories

23 programme area categories and descriptions	
Description	**Expanded description**
Infectious diseases	All diseases caused by infectious organisms, excluding tuberculosis and sexually transmitted infections
Cancers and tumours	All cancers and tumours, malignant and benign. Including those suspected or at risk of developing cancer
Blood disorders	Disorders of the blood and blood-forming systems
Endocrine, nutritional and metabolic problems (ENM)	Disorders of internal metabolism and its regulation
Mental health problems	Problems of mental health including patients with Alzheimer's syndrome
Learning disability problems	Patients where the primary issue is the problem of learning disability
Neurological system problems	Problems relating to the neurological system
Eye/vision problems	Problems relating to the eye and vision
Hearing problems	Problems relating to the ear and hearing and balance
Circulation problems	Problems relating to the heart, and the circulation of blood in central and peripheral vessels
Respiratory system problems	Problems of respiration, including tuberculosis and sleep apnoea
Dental problems	Problems due to the teeth, including preventive checks and community surveys
Gastrointestinal system problems	Problems of the gastrointestinal system
Skin problems (including burns)	Problems of the skin
Musculoskeletal system problems (excluding trauma)	Problems of the musculoskeletal system, excluding trauma
Trauma and injuries	Problems of Trauma and Injuries
Genito-urinary system disorders (except infertility)	All genito-urinary problems except for those relating to infertility
Maternity and reproductive health	Maternity and problems associated with reproduction
Neonates	Conditions of babies in the neonatal period
Poisoning	Poisoning, toxic effects and other adverse events, whether accidental or deliberate
Healthy individuals	Individuals who have no current problems, but who are involved in programmes for the prevention of illness and the promotion of good health
Social care needs	Problems related to life-management difficulty and problems related to care-provider dependency
Other	Other conditions and other congenital malformations

Source: Department of Health (2010a).

These 23 programme budget areas reflect the World Health Organization's international Classification of Diseases (ICD10). Each category represents a programme of care focused on the recipient, rather than the provider of care (Department of Health, 2010a). In England, commissioners purchase a range of different types of health care services and some services are easier to map to programme budgets than others. For example, dental services can be included under the dental problems category. More detailed information on the English NHS costing methodology can be obtained from the Department of Health (www.dh.gov.uk).

There is some dispute over the calculation and availability of cost and outcome data as these are either incomplete or out of date for some areas in England. However, 'best guess' estimation is arguably preferable to a data vacuum and, at the very least, programme budgeting resources have identified areas where data collection should be more robust. Furthermore, evidence from a recent study suggests that the use of such programme budgeting techniques offered by the Department of Health can be influential in the engagement of stakeholders (Robinson et al, 2011b). The Department of Health (England), in conjunction with other organisations, has developed a number of web-based programme budgeting tools that link budgets to outcomes measures, and these are freely available to NHS organisations. Boxes 5.2 to 5.5 outline the different tools available.

Box 5.2: The Spend and Outcomes tool: information and screenshot

The Spend and Outcomes tool has been developed by the Association of Public Health Observatories (APHO) for the Department of Health in England. This interactive tool provides a snapshot of expenditure and patient outcome data for the main programme budgeting categories. It enables comparisons to be made with the activity of other Primary Care Trusts (PCTs) nationally and allows for identification of programmes that may be driving expenditure.

The Spend and Outcomes tool is available at: www.yhpho.org.uk/resource/view. aspx?RID=49488

Figure 5.2: Screenshot of the Spend and Outcomes tool

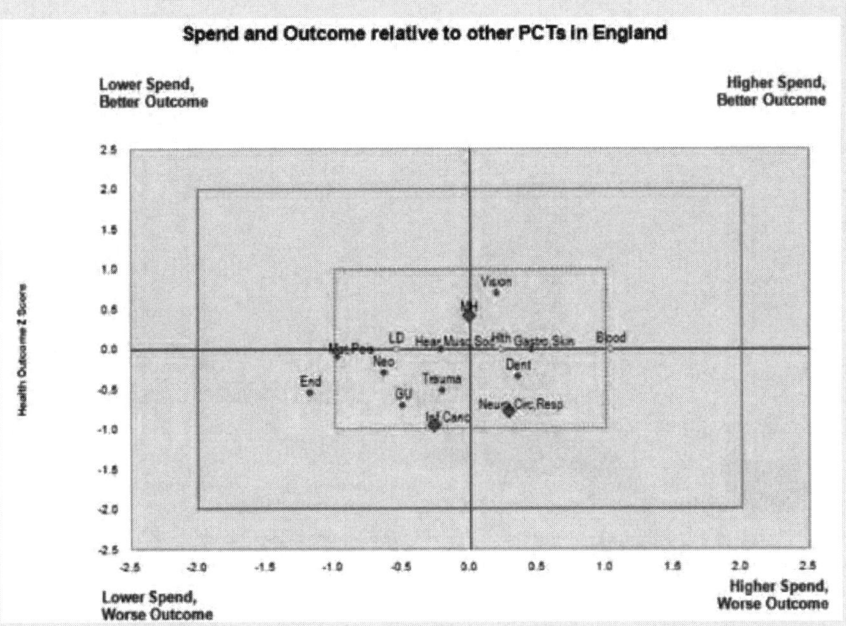

Source: Right Care (2010, p 18)

Box 5.3: Programme budgeting atlases: details and screenshot

These interactive atlases present programme budgeting expenditure data alongside clinical and health outcome indicators in a user-friendly graphical format combining maps, tables and charts. Commissioner-level programme budgeting expenditure has been linked to health outcomes, the Quality Outcome Framework (QOF) data and Hospital Episodes Statistics (HES) in the programme budgeting atlases. This tool allows commissioners to see how much is spent in each programme budget area, to compare this to other PCTs and to plot how expenditure changes over time.

The Atlases tool is available via an NHS Net connection at: nww.nchod.nhs.uk

Figure 5.3: Screenshot of the programme budgeting atlases tool

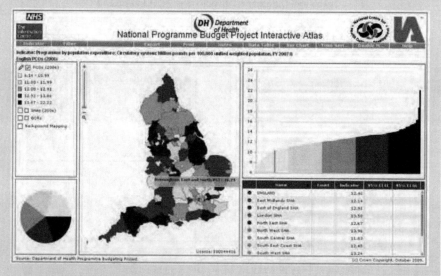

Source: Right Care (2010, p 19)

Box 5.4: NHS Comparators: information and screenshot

NHS Comparators provides quarterly inpatient activity and expenditure data by programme budget at national, strategic health authority, PCT and practice level. Prescribing expenditure and volume data linked to programme budgeting category are also available. NHS Comparators allows commissioners to track expenditure and patient outcomes over time and make timely decisions on health investment (Department of Health, 2010a).

This tool is available at: nww.nhscomparators.nhs.uk

Figure 5.4: Screenshot of the NHS Comparators tool

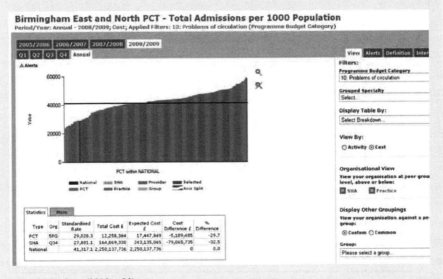

Source: Right Care (2010, p 20)

Box 5.5: Inpatient Variation Expenditure Tool (VET): information and screenshot

The Inpatient Variation Expenditure Tool (VET) allows for comparisons of inpatient admissions for high-volume disease areas. The tool can adjust expenditure to take account of population health needs. This tool helps commissioners gain further understanding of relative health expenditure, health outcomes and drivers of expenditure.

This tool is available at: www.networks.nhs.uk/nhs-networks/health-investment-network

Figure 5.5: Screenshot of the Inpatient Variation Expenditure Tool

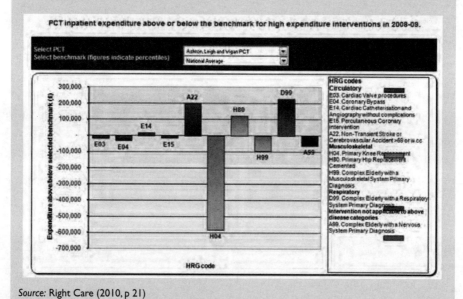

Source: Right Care (2010, p 21)

Marginal analysis

Marginal Analysis (MA) is the second phase of measurement in PBMA and begins by selecting a particular programme. The MA phase draws on economic concepts such as opportunity cost and marginal analysis to explore the assessments of costs and benefits from various health care activities involved in a particular programme area. MA is concerned with the benefit gained from the 'next unit of resource or that lost from having one unit less' (Donaldson et al, 2010). MA is usually used to assess how particular resources are utilised within a programme area and, as such, deals with issues relating to technical efficiency. However, it can also be used to explore resource allocation across programme areas (for further discussion, see Donaldson et al, 2010).

The establishment of an advisory panel with relevant stakeholders from clinical and non-clinical backgrounds is central to the MA phase. This expert panel may draw on a number of resources including: economic evaluations, needs assessments, reviews of local and national policy, and health professional and patient views. The measurement activity often involves MCDA, which enables assessment of different investment options (Donaldson et al, 2010). The panel role involves the following (Mitton and Donaldson, 2003):

- deciding on locally relevant decision-making criteria;
- focusing on the marginal benefits;
- assessing the likely impact of programme/service changes; and
- identifying areas for growth and areas for resource realisation – through reducing or decommissioning of some services.

There are a number of criticisms of the PBMA approach that recall the general drawbacks associated with MCDA. PBMA is both time and resource intensive and the actual process itself may not be cost-effective, especially if the intended efficiency savings are not realised. Further, there is often a lack of available evidence to inform the different stages of the process (Twaddle and Walker, 1995; Peacock et al, 2009; Robinson et al, 2011b). While one of the central appeals of the PBMA approach is that it provides a platform for engagement and sense of ownership for those involved in the decision-making process, gaining engagement from all relevant stakeholders can be difficult (Mitton et al, 2003). Even when stakeholders sign up to the PBMA approach and areas for change are identified, there is often reluctance from providers to give up funds for reinvestment in other areas and therefore implementation is often difficult to realise (Twaddle and Walker, 1995; Robinson et al, 2011b). In other words, like the Portsmouth scorecard and STA, PBMA is often more of a *decision-making*, rather than *implementation*, tool. The difficulties associated with implementation of priority-setting decisions are further discussed in Chapter Six.

Overall, PBMA can aid the decision-making process and provide a forum to highlight some of the tensions and issues relating to priority setting locally and can lead to greater team cohesion and enhanced stakeholder ownership of the decision-making process (Bohmer et al, 2001; Ruta et al, 2005). However, in practice, members of the public are rarely an important part of this process and this has implications for the legitimacy of decision outputs. Also PBMA, like other approaches, has tended to be applied to the allocation of resources for *new* service developments rather than the disinvestment and reallocation of resources (Mitton et al, 2003; Robinson et al, 2011a). The implications of this are that we have clear priority-setting processes for new services and interventions, but with little data in relation to the services and interventions that are already in place.

Ethical frameworks

Chapter Two outlined some of the ethical principles that may impact on health care decisions. Ethical frameworks are an attempt to combine multiple considerations into a formal framework with which to judge the merits of investment (and disinvestment) options. These frameworks typically combine a number of aspects that relate to the values of the organisation and/or wider health economy. For example, South Central Priority Setting Unit, the Oxfordshire Priorities Forum and the Healthcare Priorities Team have developed an ethical framework for their individual treatment decisions that is based on three main criteria (NHS Oxfordshire, 2010). These are:

- *Effectiveness* – evidence of benefit and possible side effects of treatment.
- *Equity* – ensure that patients suffering to a similar degree are treated equally.
- *Patient choice* – views of patient groups and individuals are considered (for further detail, see South Central Priorities support unit, 2008).

Ethical frameworks can be used in different ways. For some organisations, it may inform strategy and vision. For others, it may be used as a tool to explicitly shape resource allocation decisions. Unlike MCDA, ethical frameworks do not tend to numerically weight and/or rank the various criteria included. A recent study by Robinson et al (2011b) explored the use of ethical frameworks to inform priority setting and found that there was a gap between policy and practice. Although the policy of the priority-setting panel was to use an agreed ethical framework to support and underpin decision-making, in practice the panel made little reference to the framework within meetings. However, the study also showed that the ethical framework was used when there was disagreement between panel members or to legitimise particularly contentious decisions. These findings suggest that more clarity is required over the ways in which such tools should be applied. Robinson et al (2011b) also found that most PCT commissioners did not have formalised ethical frameworks. The absence of an explicit ethical framework does mean that many of the ethical dimensions of priority setting (and the trade-offs between them) remain largely implicit in the decision-making process. While some commissioners did not have formalised processes, they did include ethical principles in their multi-criteria scoring systems. The point here is that MCDA approaches have the capacity to include a number of different criteria that relate to different ethical standpoints.

Assessing priority-setting frameworks

There appears to be a growing interest in and usage of decision processes that involve MCDA. Although the evaluative literature on these tools remains fairly light, a number of qualified observations can be offered for those seeking to adopt and adapt such processes.

—

Consider resources

Different MCDA approaches require varying levels of complexity and analytical power. For example, the sophistication of modelling involved in the socio-technical approach goes beyond that typically associated with the Portsmouth scorecard and ethical frameworks. On the plus side, this means that decision recommendations produced are likely to be more definitive. However, it also implies the need for greater levels of resources and expertise than is associated with simpler techniques. The selection of methods should therefore reflect levels of resources and capacity as well as expertise and skills. Some priority setters may adopt a model that emphasises deliberation and engagement more than quantitative decision analysis and this may lead to selection of a more disaggregated analytical tool.

Consider information

Each of the frameworks presented here is highly dependent on the quality of information available. Although clinical opinion is suggested as a proxy for clinical evidence, this clearly has implications for the validity of decision outcomes. Overall, the message is that these tools will only be as effective as the information that is fed into them.

Consider engagement

None of the models introduced in this chapter removes the need for deliberation in the decision-making process. Indeed, the experience of users seems to be that one of the key benefits of an MCDA approach is the generation of greater (and more informed) deliberation amongst a wider group of stakeholders. In particular, the use of panel and stakeholder events can also serve to enhance understanding and potentially increase transparency and fairness. However, none of the techniques discussed, when applied in practice, has incorporated the degree of public involvement required for decisions to be either instrumentally 'correct' (ie reflecting broader social values) or legitimate in the eyes of the local public. There is, therefore, a need for such models to be accompanied by more meaningful public participation of the types discussed in Chapter Three.

Chapter summary

This chapter has introduced a number of priority-setting tools, each of which incorporates elements of MCDA. These tools and frameworks are increasingly employed by local decision-makers who value the flexibility and stakeholder engagement that they appear to facilitate. As with public involvement, engaging wider stakeholder groups in deliberative priority-setting activities can lead to: *instrumental benefits* (ie improving the quality, consistency and appropriateness of rationing decisions); *political benefits* (ie the involvement of wider stakeholder groups from across the health economy can increase democratic accountability); and *educative benefits* (ie creating a greater understanding of the complexity of decision-making and measurement aspects relating to priority setting). Further, the use of stakeholder panels provides the opportunity to develop and nurture relationships between otherwise disparate groups, and to address cultural, organisational and professional differences between these.

Up to this point, our concern has been with decision-making – that is, the process of reaching determinations over the allocation of scarce resources. However, this remains only part of the picture of priority setting and rationing in health care and there are other aspects that need to be considered. For example, the political context in which priority setters operate can determine the success or otherwise of the entire enterprise. Furthermore, the *implementation* of priority-setting decisions is as important as the decision-making process itself. Techniques such as PBMA and Portsmouth scorecards can help in identifying areas for investment and disinvestment, but often the implementation of change is much more difficult to realise. Chapters Six and Seven focus on these non-decision-making dimensions through discussion of the politics and implementation of priority setting and the leadership skills and strategies required.

Learning exercise 5.1: Multi-criteria approaches self-test

What are the main differences between approaches such as the Portsmouth scorecard, PBMA and ethical frameworks?

What are the strengths and weaknesses of MCDA when compared to other forms of decision analysis?

What factors might influence the selection of MCDA tools and processes?

SIX

The politics of priority setting

Key points covered in Chapter Six

- Without legitimacy (ie the general perception that the rationing enterprise is fair and reasonable), the most robust of decision-making processes will remain subject to attack.
- Even where decisions are based on criteria and processes that are seen to be robust, more work is required to make sure that these decisions will be accepted and enacted in full. Unless they are actually implemented, priority-setting decisions and processes will not realise the expected benefits.
- Broad notions of governance are crucial in thinking about priority setting in a context of complex, inter-organisational implementation networks.
- Interest groups have the capacity to influence priority-setting decisions and implementation. Interest groups typically sit outside of the formal decision-making process, but also often play an important role in the micro-politics of priority setting.
- The design of priority-setting processes should take account of the role of government, interest groups and the organisational and institutional contexts of both decision-making and implementation.

Introduction

Chapters Two to Five have demonstrated that there are a range of factors that can, or should, inform resource allocation decisions in health. These include considerations of ethics, process, public involvement and evidence. The challenge for decision-makers is twofold. First, they need to act on each of these requirements (ie to address ethical dimensions, to follow fair processes, to involve citizens and to make evidence-based decisions), despite limitations in the available tools and frameworks for doing so. Second, they need to combine each of these elements in ways that improve rather than confuse decision-making. Furthermore, even where decision-makers have devised decision criteria and processes that they consider to be evidence-based, inclusive and fair, more work is required if these are to be accepted and enacted in full. In order to understand how priority setting takes place, it is necessary to have an appreciation of the political and institutional realities of health care.

In traditional 'Westminster'-style political systems such as the UK, health care tends to be subject to considerable reform and regulation from central government (especially as health remains a key political issue for the electorate). Those charged with the allocation of devolved budgets, therefore, require a working knowledge of the make-up and processes of central government and their responsibilities in relation to national edicts and accountabilities. However, even in centralised systems, a plurality of groups – including professional bodies, industry, charities and academia – will endeavour to influence the terms and outcomes of priority-setting processes. Furthermore, in order to successfully *implement* decisions, priority setters require an appreciation of the complex institutional and organisational barriers to decision implementation. This chapter addresses two important themes in priority setting that challenge the conflation of priority setting and decision-making: legitimacy and implementation. Without *legitimacy* (ie the general perception that the rationing enterprise is fair and reasonable), the most robust of decision-making processes will remain subject to attack, and unless they are actually *implemented*, priority-setting decisions and processes are effectively redundant. This chapter draws on theory and research in areas of interest groups and networks, the policy process, and organisations and institutions to aid understanding and practice for those charged with managing scarcity.

Understanding policy

In order to unpack the impact that politics has on priority setting, we need to understand what we mean by policy. Policy is a term that is frequently used and yet difficult to define. This is eloquently illustrated by Cunningham (1963, p 229) who describes policy as 'rather like an elephant – you recognise it when you see it, but cannot easily define it'. Barker (1996, p 32) argues that policy is a process that 'may involve the ranking of decisions, the production of statements, the making of plans or the development of an approach'. This definition is employed here as it is particularly applicable to priority setting and resource allocation.

In this book, we deal predominantly with public policy. Dye (2001) argues that public policy is not just what governments choose to do, but also what they choose *not to do*. In other words, failure to act on an issue also constitutes policy. For example, while in opposition, the Labour Party pledged commitment to supporting older people and improving health and social care services. As a part of their 1997 manifesto, they pledged to establish a Royal Commission to explore the funding of long-term care and this was duly delivered with the creation of the Royal Commission on Long Term Care, chaired by Professor Sir Stewart Sutherland. The Royal Commission reported that the division between health and social care funding is artificial and detrimental to the care that those with long-term care needs receive in practice. Yet, as Dickinson et al (2007a) illustrate, the Labour government did not implement the recommendations of the Commission and make personal care services free, but did introduce free NHS nursing care, so that the costs of 'registered nurse time spent on providing, delegating or supervising care' would be free to everyone who needs it whether they live at home, in residential care or in a nursing home (Secretary of State for

Health, 2000, p 11). In these circumstances, the decision *not to fund* personal care is as much a policy stance as the decision *to fund* nursing care.

For the purposes of this book, then, policy is a process that incorporates not only those things that governments do, but also those things that they choose not to do. Policy is clearly, then, a fundamental part of priority setting and rationing. Although at a national level, government policy determines what the NHS should and should not do, governments have tended to avoid formal responsibility for deciding which services should be denied to patients. In England and Wales in recent years, this position has been somewhat modified with the setting up of the National Institute for Health and Clinical Excellence (NICE), and through the legal mandate enshrined in the NHS Constitution, which:

> establishes the principles and values of the NHS in England … sets out rights to which patients, public and staff are entitled, and pledges which the NHS is committed to achieve, together with responsibilities which the public, patients and staff owe to one another to ensure that the NHS operates fairly and effectively. All NHS bodies and private and third sector providers supplying NHS services are required by law to take account of this Constitution in their decisions and actions. (Department of Health, 2010b, p 2)

Although governments remain reluctant to deal with the minutiae of rationing, they are often less hesitant in shaping the behaviours of those who do. The NHS, for example, has been accused of being a 'centrist' system subject to frequent reform and regulation from central government (Dickinson et al, 2007b). For this reason, it has often been argued that local health care organisations have little autonomy over the types of rationing decisions that they are able to make, and, in recent times, this has been notably true in relation to Primary Care Trusts (PCTs) (Smith et al, 2010). As a result of this central involvement, decision-makers do not always have the latitude to make the decisions that we might expect. Buse et al (2005), therefore, argue that it is impossible to understand health policy without considering politics, and there are many potential levels at which politics has an impact on rationing and priority setting. In recent years, there have been a number of attempts to 'depoliticise' decision-making – for example, through the work of NICE – and these efforts often use technical and scientific approaches to rationing. Klein (2010) terms these attempts a 'technocratic chastity belt', while acknowledging that in practice this does not remove politics from priority setting or rationing.

The commissioning agenda in the English NHS – involving the devolvement of much resource allocation responsibilities to PCTs – has implications for the priority-setting function. However, there is no 'national template' of how PCTs (or their successor commissioners) set about the task, or any guidance about how prioritisation criteria are defined, weighted or applied (Klein, 2010, p 393). Furthermore, although formal responsibility is given to PCTs, the government reserves the right to intervene where it objects to the decisions reached (Harding,

2005). This picture – in which local processes are subject to macro-political intervention – is common across health care systems (see eg Yeo et al, 1999).

The equivocal, inconsistent and occasionally misleading role played by governments in local processes of priority setting can damage the latter's legitimacy in the eyes of local stakeholders. This in turn creates difficulties for leaders of priority setting who are required to respond to government demands while protecting the integrity of local processes. The forms of leadership required in this situation are the subject of Chapter Seven. For the purposes of this chapter, it is important to note that even when resource allocation responsibilities are devolved to local decision-makers, this is rarely carried out without government involvement, and therefore the extent of local autonomy in decision-making is open to question.

Understanding institutions and organisations

Like policy, although we often use the terms organisation and institution, these are rather less frequently defined. Further, even when these are defined, there is often little in the way of a clear distinction between the two terms. Organisations can be characterised as the social means through which groups pursue collective goals, and these normally have a boundary that separates the entity from its environment. Clearly, this is a wide-ranging definition and becomes even more so when we consider that organisations might be formally structured (like a hospital or a university), but may also be less formal (like a local youth or football club).

According to Child (1988), organisational structures can be broken down into the following components:

* *Basic structure* – the formal allocation of people and resources to the tasks that have to be done and the mechanisms for their coordination.
* *Operating mechanisms* – standing orders, operating procedures, control procedures, performance standards and review.
* *Decision mechanisms* – procedures for information gathering and processing, specification of decision processes, rules and audit.

This analysis is important as dysfunction in the structure might lead to delayed or poor-quality decision-making. If we consider priority setting as part of the decision mechanism, it is important that it is carefully integrated with the other two components of organisational structure. Without this type of integration, information might not be transferred on time to the right people and decision makers may therefore become segmented and uncoordinated. Other consequences of poor alignment can be the overloading of some decision-making roles and an absence of procedures for evaluating decisions to ensure consistency.

Institutions are defined by Berger and Luckmann (1966) as the structure and mechanisms of social order and cooperation that govern the behaviours of a group of individuals. Key points here are that institutions have a social purpose and are formed to enforce rules and govern cooperative behaviours between individuals. Some formal organisations are identified as institutions and are intentionally created by groups – the NHS is a good example of this. In the case of examples like the NHS, these are conscious decisions made in order to create appropriate structures for particular purposes (ie providing health services to the English population).

However, other institutions go beyond the conscious intentions of the individuals involved. Again, the NHS is a good example. As a mechanism of cooperation, the institution of the NHS has a number of formal organisations such as hospitals, mental health trusts and so on, but the NHS also contains more informal institutions of social order. As Glasby et al (2007b, p 3) argue, the NHS is also a key British institution that is crucial to patients and to the public alike – both in terms of the services it offers and the values it embodies. Indeed, in a time of rapid change, the NHS may even be seen as central to our identity – if we asked the general public to identify a key symbol of Britishness, the NHS would be likely to emerge as a key national asset and symbol. As a result of this, it is entirely appropriate that the NHS should work to priorities and within parameters set by elected politicians, and that it should be accountable to our elected representatives for the quality of its services and its use of taxpayers' money. As discussed in Chapter Two, the NHS is an institution in the sense that it embodies the values and beliefs of universality and access to services regardless of an individual's ability to pay for these. It embodies a sense of social solidarity that reflects a strain of broader civic culture and identity.

Traditionally, institutions of government have been associated with particular functions (see Table 6.1), but the degree to which these are clearly understood or have played out in rationing practices is questionable. We might think of the organisational in the sense of the 'structure' of relationships. In doing so, thinking about the organisational might involve mapping out the committees, membership structures and reporting relationships of priority-setting processes. Institutions, on the other hand, might be thought of in terms of the 'practices' of priority-setting processes. The institutional context is therefore comprised of procedures and practices, local rituals, the types of norms that are viewed as appropriate and how individuals and groups 'perform'. For the purposes of this discussion, it is important to note the structuring effects that institutional norms and rituals can have on priority setting through the 'rules constraining the actions of participating actors' (Schedler and Glastra, 2001, p 690). In other words, without a compatible

Table 6.1: Institutions of government and their functions: a traditional view

Institution of government	Function
Legislature	Representation
Executive	Policy formulation
Bureaucracy	Policy implementation
Judiciary	Dispute resolution

environment, priority setting will go against the institutional grain, and will therefore encounter resistance.

Interest groups

As well as being constrained by governmental, organisational and institutional factors, priority-setting processes are invariably subject to interest group lobbying and involvement. Even though the UK has a relatively centralised health system, there is still a plurality of groups who might seek to influence the terms and outcomes of priority-setting processes. The term 'interest group' refers to non-state actors – voices from 'civil society' – sometimes referred to as 'pressure groups'. These tend to be groups and/or organisations rather than individuals, who operate at a range of levels from local and regional through to national and international. These are voluntary groups who tend to be goal-oriented in the sense that they have a particular aim in mind. Interest groups seek to influence, but they do not – at least initially – seek formal power, although there are some examples of interest groups who have developed to achieve formal power over time (Buse et al, 2005).

Grant (1984) distinguishes between sectional and cause, and between insider and outsider, groups. Sectional groups seek to protect and enhance the cause of the members of society or the particular group they stand for. So, for example, professional representation bodies or trade unions are examples of sectional groups. By contrast, cause groups seek to advance a particular issue and are typically open to everyone that supports that cause. Examples of cause groups include those that focus on particular diseases, the environment and so on.

The distinction between sectional and cause groups is important in the context of health care rationing as sectional groups often have a degree of power over decisions and their implementation. As Buse et al (2005) identify, sectional groups often stand for producer interests (eg doctors, nurses etc), whilst cause groups stand for consumer interests (eg particular disease groups). This is a helpful heuristic to use in thinking about interest groups, but the distinction is sometimes less clear-cut than we would imagine and groups may move between being sectional and cause groups over time. Whether groups are insider or outsider groups depends on the proximity of these groups to the decision-making process. Insiders are seen as having a right of say in the processes of policymaking and are invited to sit with decision-makers and talk about issues and may be invited to sit on committees and so on. Outsiders either reject a close relationship with policymakers or else are not considered by these to be a legitimate part of the decision-making process. Again, though, groups may find that they move between these broad categories at different times.

So why is it important that we think about interest groups and the various forms that they might take? The interplay of interest group agendas is nowhere more significant than in health care:

—

The existence of interest group considerations may ... introduce additional constraints into the priority setting process, such as requiring that a certain proportion of available funds are spent in particular areas or on specific programmes; or that policy changes do not alienate powerful groups. (Goddard et al, 2006, p 85)

Peterson (1999) argues that interest groups play a number of functions in society and these are set out in Box 6.1. From this it is clear that interest groups play an array of different roles and are important in terms of the social institution of the NHS and resource allocation decisions. There are many examples of the influence of interest groups in health care and their impacts on rationing decisions. Often these will not reach the attention of the general public and were these influences to take place through insider groups and 'normal processes' of government and governance, we might not have cause to notice these interactions. However, where these are new issues or come from outsider groups, there may be more media attention and cause for the general public to be more aware of the role of interest groups.

Box 6.1: The functions of interest groups

- *Participation* – this is a way for citizens to claim a voice around public issues.
- *Representation* – interest groups are a way of gaining wider ranges of views than would otherwise be incorporated by governments.
- *Political education* – involvement in interest groups is a way of learning about the political process.
- *Motivation* – interest groups drawing attention to issues can motivate governments to take issues seriously.
- *Monitoring* – interest groups increasingly have a role in monitoring the performance of the government.
- *Provision* – interest groups are involved in the delivery of services (with or without government funding).

Learning exercise 6.1: Understanding interest groups

Consider priority setting in your health care economy. How many different local interest groups can you think of? How would you classify these? Are they sectional or cause groups; insider or outsider?

Many of the examples of interest groups and priority setting that have gained attention in recent years have been in relation to decisions on drug treatments. The drug Herceptin and its use in early stage cancer is one such example. Following the publicity that surrounded research reported in an academic journal, Herceptin became demanded in many countries around the world despite the fact that it was unlicensed for treatment of early breast cancer and the drug's manufacturer had not yet submitted data for the approval of the drug (Piccart-Gebhart et al, 2005; Romond et al, 2005). Subsequently, many governments bypassed their own normal processes for approving drugs or funding treatments. For example, in France, the normal procedures for approval were bypassed (*The Lancet*, 2005) and several Canadian provinces fast-tracked approval (Kondro and Sibbald, 2005).

In the UK, the process of assessment was also accelerated under considerable media and political attention. Ferner and McDowell (2006) illustrate how patients and their support groups, the media, the pharmaceutical industry, and politicians all exerted pressure to bypass established processes of technology coverage decision-making in order that Herceptin would be made available. These authors argue that the 'role of NICE is critically important to the rational distribution of NHS funds', and that 'in an ideal world the [drug] appraisal process would be insulated, and be seen to be insulated, from external financial, political and emotional pressures' (Ferner and McDowell, 2006, p 1270). That this was not the case in practice testifies to the impact that a campaign of interest group lobbying can have in resource allocation. These pressures again recall the dual perspectives on priority setting introduced in the introduction – that of the rationalist versus pluralist – inasmuch as decision outcomes reflected a pluralistic process of politics as much as they did the application of evidence and decision analysis.

In analysing the relative influence of interest groups over the decision-making process, it is useful to draw on the concept of policy framing. 'Frames' are essentially ways of understanding a policy issue in order to provide 'conceptual coherence, a direction for action, a basis for persuasion, and a framework for the collection and analysis of data' (Rein and Schön, 1993, p 153). Different groups will seek to assert or impose their preferred policy frame so that decisions are taken according to their underlying perspectives. Or, in other words groups will seek to frame issues in the most efficacious manner so they can so that they gain the buy-in of stakeholders. Returning to the example of Herceptin, a study of media representation of the debates about this drug in Australia (MacKenzie et al, 2008) looked at the different ways the drug and its impact were framed. This study found that 'the dominant discourse across the news coverage was that Herceptin was a "wonder drug" made unaffordable to the majority of women with HER2 breast cancer by government indifference, labyrinthine bureaucracy and unacceptable, financial parsimony' (MacKenzie et al, 2008, p 307). Similar patterns can be found in reporting of rationing of Avastin, a drug for patients with advanced bowel cancer. One such newspaper headline ran 'Avastin prolongs life but drug is too expensive for NHS patients, says NICE' (Pidd, 2010). Thus, this story is framed in such a way as to gloss over concerns regarding quality of life and/or opportunity cost.

—

The micro-politics of priority setting

Whether formulated as a committee, a network or a panel, priority-setting bodies usually meet in a face-to-face setting to discharge the decision-making function, with the support of pre-reading and other information deemed relevant. The reality of ethical pluralism, data shortages and vested interests means that subsequent decisions will be shaped by the exchange of views of those involved. In other words, *deliberation* at the meeting is an inevitable and important influence on decision outputs (van Stokkom, 2005). Therefore, it is important in understanding priority setting to explore how these processes work, and in a normative sense to think about how such deliberations *should* proceed. A number of recent studies involve real-time observation of priority-setting meetings (eg Singer et al, 2000; Williams and Bryan, 2007a; Russell and Greenhalgh, 2009). These studies suggest that deliberative elements of decision processes tend to be less well articulated and less transparent than evidence-generating components.

Conducting deliberations behind 'closed doors' enables decision-makers to acknowledge the vagueness and uncertainty surrounding decisions while at the same time projecting an appearance of certainty and precision to an outside audience (Chambers, 2004). In these deliberations, a range of factors can influence decisions and much will depend on patterns of dominance and subordination that are played out between those in attendance. In a study of local technology coverage committees, Williams (2009) identified four distinct ways in which decisions were framed by participants and noted that these were in tension and competed for prominence. The four frames were:

- *Frame One – Pursuit of clinical effectiveness.* This was cited as the most important consideration and constituted the main area of expertise within committees.
- *Frame Two – Controlling costs of introduction.* This was the second most evident frame adopted and reflected concern over the likely impact of decisions on budgets. This was often considered to be the main priority of specific committee members – for example, those with responsibilities for commissioning and/ or finance.
- *Frame Three – Achieving value for money and disinvesting in inefficient technologies.* This was essentially a peripheral frame that was cited more as an ambition than as an actual guiding framework. It is this frame that would privilege information such as health technology assessment and cost-effectiveness analysis.
- *Frame Four – Inclusion and accountability.* This was mentioned only in passing, and by a minority of respondents. With a few exceptions, the decision-making bodies studied did not see patient and/or public involvement as central to their work.

Although frames one, two and three privilege use of information, the nature of this information was different in each case. In the case of the 'clinical effectiveness' frame, expert opinion served as a supplement or substitute for published evidence.

In general, there was a combination of frames invoked at any given time. Data from observations suggest that the pursuit of clinical effectiveness and 'managed introduction' (frames one and two) superseded 'technology assessment and appraisal' (frame three), although these were often confused or apparently in competition. Overall, the widespread pre-eminence of clinical effectiveness as a driver of decisions reflects the dominance of a biomedical frame over one of decision analysis informed by consideration of efficiency.

Russell and Greenhalgh (2009) also employ the concept of frames in a case study of a priority-setting body in the NHS. They note the power attributed to 'numbers' (as proxies for 'facts') in the persuasion strategies adopted by those taking part in decision-making, with other data – for example, the experiential wisdom of practitioners – treated as comparatively peripheral. Thus, the institutional setting will have a great degree of influence over what kinds of evidence are seen as valid within particular priority-setting environments. Box 6.2 provides a further example, this time within the context of 'joined-up' priority setting between health and social care agencies.

Box 6.2: Joined-up health and social care priority setting in England

The notion of collaboration has been central to health and social care policy for some time and it is widely accepted that health and social care organisations need to work together in order to deliver services effectively (Glasby and Dickinson, 2008). If this is the case, then it is important that priority setting is carried out in a joined-up manner.

However, there are a number of barriers that need to be addressed. For example, the NHS approach to nationally collected tax-based revenue is in marked contrast to the picture that has developed in social care – most notably in relation to the expanded role afforded to local government, but also in the prominence of means testing, co-payments and devolvement of budgets to individual service users. The danger is that the mismatch in decision-making structures and financing strategies leads to a lack of equivalence in terms of the roles and remits of collaborating priority setters.

A second difference relates to accessing services. In social care, priority setting is largely embedded in needs assessment criteria, and rationing takes place through the application of funding thresholds to these needs-based categories of eligibility. In the NHS, the expectation is that no patient with legitimate health care needs should be denied care irrespective of condition severity (despite concerns over the plausibility of this expectation). Therefore, the strategies employed in social care – denying services to those with lower levels of need and setting user charges at different levels in different localities – are less plausible in health.

A third area of difference relates to the role of evidence. As we have seen, in health care there have been strong calls for priority setting to be informed by quantitative decision analysis (Williams, 1998). By contrast, successful interventions in social care are more likely to be linked to notions such as lived experience, adaptation and empowerment, which are inherently difficult to codify and measure (Dickinson, 2008). Finally, the political contexts and accountability structures facing decision-makers are considerably different in each sector.

While overcoming these obstacles entirely may not be feasible, at least in the short term, there are a number of factors that may help to lessen their impact. For example, there is recent precedent in terms of pooling budgets and this may help to reduce some of the asymmetries of decision-making in health and social care systems. Further alignment of funding models may also result from the trend in health towards both individualised budgets and greater levels of patient co-payment for selected interventions.

With regard to service access, it is not clear that the barriers to integration posed by the different models of health and social care can be overcome without, in effect, one side adopting the other's model.

The different mechanisms for rationing care and the types of 'evidence' privileged in each context pose considerable difficulties. However, in relation to the role of evidence, both parties could benefit from greater dialogue – social care through exploration of the potential benefits of investing in population-level evidence generation, and health through the development of less narrow measures of service 'outcomes' and a more sophisticated appreciation of the impact on service users and their families.

Despite differing political contexts, what is common across both these environments is that priority setting is more than simply a technical exercise.

Source: Williams et al (2011a).

Implementation

As we have already suggested, resource allocation decisions will have little impact unless they are implemented in practice. The issue of the 'implementation gap' has been a key consideration of social policy academics and policymakers alike for some time. The challenges facing rationers when seeking to implement policy decisions can be illustrated through the application of Matland's (1995) ambiguity–conflict model (see Table 6.2). According to Matland, approaches to implementation should reflect the extent of ambiguity and conflict surrounding a policy. Where these measures are both *low* (ie there is clarity over aims and little or no disagreement between those involved), a rational, linear approach to implementation might reasonably be adopted. In these circumstances, implementation is characterised as 'administrative' and depends in large part on

Table 6.2: Matland's (1995) ambiguity–conflict model

	Low conflict	High conflict
Low ambiguity	Administrative implementation	Political implementation
High ambiguity	Experimental implementation	Symbolic implementation

the availability of resources. In conditions of *low ambiguity and high conflict* (ie where the aims of policy are clear, but disputed), the approach to implementation will require some exercise of either power or negotiation – for example, through sanctions or incentives for compliance. In cases of *low conflict and high ambiguity*, policies are likely to be implemented in an experimental fashion with emphasis, at least in the short term, on learning rather than results. Finally, policies marked by *high ambiguity and high conflict* are likely to be dependent on coalitions of actors at the local level for their implementation, with reduced scope for central control.

As resource allocation decisions often involve the removal or withholding of potentially beneficial interventions, we might assume that they will invariably be surrounded by significant levels of conflict as those who 'lose out' (either as patients, producers or professionals) will object. As we have seen, it is also typical for priority-setting activities to lack clarity of purpose – as multiple objectives, principles and influences are brought to bear on decisions. Such decisions frequently fall into the category of high ambiguity and high conflict and this goes some way towards explaining why the 'nettle' of explicit rationing is rarely grasped in full. Instead, compromises are sought and definitive statements of purpose are avoided in order to maintain a fragile peace between stakeholders at the local and national levels. Indeed, NICE can be seen as an example of how attempts to reduce ambiguity (by adopting clear decision criteria) can increase conflict (Syrett, 2003).

So how does this manifest in practice? All too often, local priority setters are given insufficient clarity from political overseers with respect to the aims and criteria of rationing (Klein et al, 1996) and, as we saw in Chapter Three, this shortfall is not currently mitigated by public engagement. Without a clearer conception of aims, decisions (and their implementation) are more likely to be influenced by bargaining between local interest groups, making power an important consideration in the implementation phase (Milewa and Barry, 2005). Decision-makers may also experience resistance and blockages from within the front-line and implementing organisations, as any priority-setting function or process will be located in a broader decision, delivery and performance management system and this context will therefore impact upon the success or otherwise of its operations and outputs. If the implementation of priority-setting decisions is to shift from the bottom-right quadrant of Matland's matrix to the top-left quadrant, then the challenges of ambiguity and conflict will need to be addressed.

Governance and performance

We contend that the factors introduced in this chapter – government, organisations, institutions and implementation barriers – all point to the need for effective *governance* of resource allocation and for attention to be paid to the *performance* of priority setting. At this point, it is perhaps helpful to think of the framework of performance developed by Jon McKenzie (2001) as a way of teasing out the difference between structures and practices. Kershaw (2006, p 30) argues that in recent decades we have seen the emergence of 'performative societies' where 'the human is increasingly constituted through performance'. McKenzie (2001) suggests that there are three predominant types of performance – organisational (efficiency), technological (effectiveness) and cultural (efficacy) – and proposes a theory of performance that is a confluence of these distinct forms of performance. Efficiency is considered as a means to utilise the minimum inputs possible to obtain a required quantity and quality of outputs. Efficiency, therefore, might be represented as '*doing the thing right*'. Effectiveness refers to the extent to which an organisation has a programme of activities that will deliver its established goals or intended aims; effectiveness, therefore, is about '*doing the right thing*' to deliver the outcomes it has determined (or has been set). Efficacy, on the other hand, relates to the extent to which an organisation is perceived to be achieving outcomes that are valued by its main stakeholders. Efficacy, then, is about '*according with conceptions of rightness*' in the eyes of service users, their carers, members of the public and their democratic representatives. Efficacy, therefore, clearly incorporates consideration of the types of institutions that are influential in terms of particular stakeholder groups and settings.

According to McKenzie, performance is not a simple, coherent and stable concept; rather, it is dynamic, responding to changes in dominant socio-cultural forces. Thus, the parameters of 'high' performance will alter according to the values and norms prevalent in social, political and organisational systems. The implication of this is that it is insufficient for priority-setting processes to simply be efficient or effective – they must also be efficacious – that is, appeal to institutional values (for an analysis of PCT commissioning also using this framework, see Dickinson et al, 2010). In other words, priority-setting processes must be seen to incorporate the values of various stakeholder groups in order to be seen as legitimate. It is not just about making the 'right' decision; it is about making the decision in the 'right' way, taking into account the right sorts of values and opinions. As we have already suggested, this is not an easy thing to achieve given the many different ethical standpoints that underpin health services. Yet this also suggests why it is that even when robust processes are in place to collect and analyse evidence, they may not make decisions that are accepted or implemented.

Poor decision-making is perhaps one reason why there has been such attention to notions of corporate governance in recent years. In the 1980s and 1990s, a series of corporate scandals (eg World Corp, Enron and Arthur Anderson) focused attention on how organisations operate and make decisions (Knights and O'Leary,

2005). However, the issue of poor decision-making was considered less in terms of the specific decisions made, than with how individuals were allowed to make these decisions and whether they and their organisations were subsequently held accountable. A series of high-profile business scandals have led to a focus on the notion of organisations achieving 'good corporate governance'. Peck and Dickinson (2008, p 60) define governance as the 'mechanisms that legitimise authority, accountability, policies and procedures in organisations – or in the relationships between organisations – within the social and political environment in which they operate'. Yet what is meant by 'good' governance is less than clear, and, in recent years, a large literature has sprung up that attempts to set out what is meant by this (see Box 6.3). Whilst there are some differences between these definitions, there are some common themes in terms of direction, control, values and accountability.

> ## Box 6.3: Definitions of corporate governance
>
> 'A system by which an organisation is directed and controlled' (The Committee on the Financial Aspect of Corporate Governance and Gee and Co Ltd, 1992; known as the 'Cadbury Report').
>
> 'The structure through which the objectives of the company are set, and the means of attaining those objectives and monitoring performance are determined' (Organisation for Economic Co-operation and Development, 2004).
>
> 'To ensure an organisation fulfils its purpose, achieves its intended outcomes for citizens and service users, and operates in an effective, efficient and ethical manner' (Independent Commission, 2004; known as the 'Langlands Principles').

However, it is not just a concern with bad decision-making and corporate scandals that has focused attention on governance. Lynn et al (2001, p 1) argue that this recent focus on governance is due to public policies increasingly being delivered 'through complicated webs of states, regions ... non-profit organizations, collaborations, networks, partnerships and other means for the control and coordination of dispersed activities'.

As well as being upwardly accountable to government and national policy bodies, local decision-makers must therefore also engage a plethora of local stakeholders and citizens, and 'manage the message' of priority setting in a difficult economic climate. These complicated webs have to achieve public purposes in a context where traditional accountability to elected national politicians and local councillors is increasingly supplemented by the likes of appointed boards, neighbourhood councils and the co-option of service users. Governance of these 'webs' is often discharged by deliberately hybrid groups drawn from many sources in order to give legitimacy to decisions. This can be seen, for example, in the attempts to bring together stakeholders as part of processes such as accountability for reasonableness

(A4R) and programme budgeting and marginal analysis (PBMA) (see Chapters Two and Five, respectively, for more detail). While effective corporate governance is important, these wider forms of governance are perhaps more important in thinking about the nature of priority setting in health care.

Far from being a purely technical or procedural process, priority setting requires political acumen and skills in relationship management and coalition building so that 'tough choices' can be taken and implemented without undermining trust in health care institutions. The extent to which such processes are managed will therefore be important in determining the success of any priority-setting endeavour (this issue is revisited in Chapter Seven). An implication is that although much of the priority-setting literature and activity has recently focused on the efficiency and effectiveness of processes and the types of approaches set out in the previous two chapters, this does not negate the need for legitimacy, and arguably more attention should be paid to the wider issues of the efficacy of these processes.

If we think of governance in a broader sense than simply corporate governance, we might understand it as a process of:

- securing agreement on a programme of action among a diversity of actors/ organisations;
- redistributing the capacity of actors/organisations to interpret decisions according to their own values; and
- gaining acceptance that resulting actions are legitimate (Contandripoulos et al, 2004).

This understanding of governance requires us to look beyond single organisations towards the wider decision-making and implementation contexts.

Although it is often suggested that good governance should lead to better organisational performance, the evidence to support this is limited. From a review of the literature, Skelcher et al (2004, p 14) conclude: 'the theoretical connections between governance arrangements and organisational performance are poorly supported by empirical evidence'. The familiar view of the priority-setting committee depicts their function as *instrumental*. In other words, they are there to make decisions, to engage in deliberation and to conciliate where conflict arises. This is the view reflected in much of the prescriptive guidance on the role of boards more generally: they are to be measured, on this account, by the extent to which they efficiently and effectively discharge the decision-making function (Simon, 1997 [1945]). This is the perception of boards commonly held by the public, by many policymakers and often by priority-setting panels themselves (Robinson et al, 2011b).

Another view is that boards (and priority-setting bodies) perform other unspoken organisational roles – that is, those that do not appear on the agenda and yet are carried out in the course of members being in the same place and speaking or remaining silent according to certain conventions. In this view, boards are arenas in which those present tell stories about who they collectively are, sustain culture, organise shared emotions, sustain loyalty and conciliate over social relations in conflicts. This supports the claim that the work of boards is primarily *symbolic* (Huff, 1988; Schwartzman, 1989). When applied to priority setting, this again implies the need to take account of the importance of *efficacy*.

As Peck and Dickinson (2008) argue, good governance is seen to exist when boards effectively undertake the limited instrumental tasks available to them and do so in a manner that symbolises the collective and consensual approach to the delivery of public services in which they are involved. In the provision of public services by networks of organisations, good governance has to both *deliver legitimacy* (by engaging the appropriate range of stakeholders) and *perform legitimacy* (by building cohesion and commitment). Poor governance, therefore, will do neither. Skelcher et al (2004, p 14) conclude, 'it is easier to establish the implications of governance arrangements for democratic performance than for organisational performance'; that is, it is easier to show that a specific form of governance has contributed to symbolic performance (such as being seen to be legitimate) than it has to instrumental performance (such as actually achieving targets).

This focus on the symbolic role of decision-making bodies has a number of implications for priority setters (Cornforth, 2003). In particular it suggests the importance of:

- being clear when you are discussing governance with organisational partners that you are all talking about the same thing;
- being realistic about the limits of the instrumental impact of your governance arrangements; and
- being aware of the potential – both positive but also negative – of the symbolic impact of these arrangements.

In terms of priority setting, these prescriptions go beyond simply engaging with technical approaches and are concerned with how these connect to the wider structures of governance with which priority-setting processes and systems are situated.

Learning exercise 6.2: Understanding institutions and governance

Think about the ways in which priority setting operates in your locality. What are the important organisations and institutions that have influence on these processes? How are these connected and governed? If this is a board, which of Cornforth's perspectives on organisational governance do you think this reflects? Share your thoughts with a colleague and see if you have the same perspective.

Implications for priority setting

Although there is a substantial literature on health care organisations and institutions, relatively little is known about the specific implications of these for local-level priority setting. As a result, much of the responsibility for designing local systems has been left to local organisations themselves. This potentially leads to significant variation in relation to factors such as: the remit and 'clout' of priority-setting bodies; the stated roles and responsibilities of individual participants; and the linkage between determinations reached and actual resource allocation processes within and across organisations. The risk is that there is a failure to securely embed priority setting within organisational (and inter-organisational) systems (Williams and Bryan, 2007b).

In designing suitable systems, Weiss (1979, p 428) emphasises the need for a 'well defined decision situation'. Important requirements of such a situation include:

- agreement as to what the decision options are;
- specification of what evidence and considerations are permissible for consideration; and
- confirmation of whether or not the decision-making committee considers the full implications and impact of their decisions.

However, issues of efficacy and legitimacy require decision-makers to situate their processes in a wider context of: governmental requirements; organisational and institutional cultures; and complex implementation systems. Possible leadership responses to these factors are explored in Chapter Seven.

Box 6.4: Convening a priority-setting committee: areas to consider

What types of decisions are considered by the committee?
- Individual cases.
- Availability of new treatments.
- Allocation of additional resources.
- Allocation of core spend.

What organisational and geographical remit will the committee have?
- Single organisation.
- All commissioning organisations.
- All health care organisations.
- Health and other (eg social care) organisations.

How will committee decisions be fed into subsequent resource allocation?
- Decisions will be formally binding on all contributing organisations.
- Decisions will form recommendations to guide resource allocation.
- Decisions will constitute information to support actual resource allocation decisions.

What are the roles and expectations of committee members?
- Committee members will be expected to bring specific expertise to bear on decisions.
- Committee members will be expected to advocate on behalf of specific user/population groups.
- Committee members will be expected to adopt the committee's interests and to act on behalf of the overall population served by the prioritisation process.
- Committee members are expected to represent the interests of their organisation and/ or sector.

How will information be generated and analysed?
- What specific information resources will be required?
- How will this information be fed into decision-making?
- What data analysis skills are required by individual decision-makers?

Learning exercise 6.3: Designing a decision-making body

Imagine you are setting up a priority-setting committee in your local area. Using the guidance set out in Box 6.4, design your ideal committee. Consider the following aspects:

- What are the implications of this design?
- What tradeoffs have you made and will these have an implication in terms of the implementation of these decisions?

Chapter summary

So far, we have argued that looking 'inwards' at decision-making criteria and processes is insufficient if our aim is to implement acceptable and efficacious priority setting. In this chapter, we have started to reflect on wider determinants and the impact of these in terms of legitimacy and implementation. We argue that without legitimacy (ie the general perception that the rationing enterprise is fair and reasonable), even the most robust of decision-making processes will remain open to attack, and that unless decisions are actually implemented, then priority-setting processes are effectively redundant. Using McKenzie's terminology, we argue that prescriptions for priority setting have tended to focus on *efficiency* and *effectiveness* at the expense of *efficacy* – and this may help to explain why many attempts to implement explicit decision-making approaches have had limited success. Without a more concerted intervention into structures and cultures of *governance*, and greater attention to the *performance* of priority setting, such experiences are likely to continue. In Chapter Seven, we consider the role of leadership in addressing these constraining factors in priority setting.

SEVEN

Leadership in priority setting

Key points covered in Chapter Seven

- Resource scarcity in health care can be seen as a 'wicked' problem requiring specific leadership responses. However, the literature on leadership in priority setting is underdeveloped.
- Leadership functions in priority setting go beyond narrow models of governance and should reflect the relational nature of governance in complex systems.
- Leaders should engage in sensemaking in support of the priority-setting enterprise.
- Leaders should develop political skills in order to protect priority-setting processes from being undermined.
- Leaders should seek to align values with the deployment of resources and the demands of government, organisations and institutions.
- Clinical leadership is important to effective priority setting.

Introduction

In the last chapter, we argued for the importance to successful priority setting of having compatible political and institutional contexts, and therefore the need to move beyond reductive approaches that focus exclusively on *decision-making*. Unless decision-making is aligned with wider systems of governance and supported by effective relationship and profile management, rationing outcomes may not be achieved. This chapter considers the role played by individuals in responding to these challenges. In any resource allocation process, individuals will be required to take responsibility for tasks such as: facilitating deliberation; resolving conflicts; engaging with media and other stakeholders; negotiating with government; managing public expectations; ensuring implementation; performance management and so on. Therefore, ensuring that these and other elements of successful priority setting take place requires both management and *leadership*. As this has been largely neglected in the priority-setting literature this chapter draws lessons and learning from the broader leadership literature. In particular, we discuss the relevance to priority setting of conceptions of leadership as relational, as political astuteness and as involving sensemaking.

Terminology

In recent years, the notion of 'strong leadership' has become firmly embedded within every walk of life and it is generally accepted that strong leadership should bring about significant improvements in everything from football teams, to child safeguarding, to economic stability. Yet, despite these beliefs, we know surprisingly little about what leadership is and how it works. Although one of the most researched areas of the last 50 years, leadership remains contested, under-theorised and reliant on a few popular views (Bolden and Gosling, 2006). In seeking to define what leadership is and how it might be studied, Peck and Dickinson (2009) note that the study of leadership has moved through a series of stages, each of which reflect the popular social and cultural beliefs and values of the period. These are summarised in Table 7.4. What Table 7.1 suggests is that how we view leadership depends on the prevailing culture and social environment (as well as one's place; Mabey and Finch-Lees, 2008). Therefore, definitions of leadership depend on the context within which it is enacted, making immutable definitions not only unattainable, but also undesirable (Gemmill and Oakley, 1992). However, despite this lack of definitional clarity, leadership is increasingly considered central to processes of change in health care. Hartley and Benington (2010, p 3), for example, note that 'better leadership is seen as central to improving the quality of health care and the improvement of organisational processes'.

Table 7.1: Summary of major approaches to leadership

Approach	Emphasis	Development implications
Great Man	Personal Traits	Few – leaders are born, not made. Assumes that the leadership characteristics of the individual are innate and that context had little influence therefore.
Situational/ personal-situational	Context dependence	Suggests that leaders can develop interpersonal skills to some degree, and the importance of developing different leadership approaches in different contexts.
Psychological profiling	Psychological traits	Limited development of the interpersonal dimensions of leadership. Relies heavily on an individualistic perspective.
Behavioural	Actions appropriate to followership	Draws attention to the identity of leaders as relational rather than individual. Suggests importance of intrapersonal development.
Transformational	Relationship between leader and followers	Leadership understood as 'a function of a community not a result derived from an individual deemed to be objectively superhuman' (Grint, 2005b, p 2). Suggests importance of development of inter- and intrapersonal dimensions.
Constitutive	Sensemaking	Recognises that leadership is constituted in interpersonal exchanges (ie someone is a leader if they are considered as such by others) and also as part of broader social and cultural contexts. Draws attention to the dependence of leadership on 'followership' and therefore the need to develop inter- and intrapersonal dimensions.

Source: Peck and Dickinson (2008, p 24).

The role of leadership in priority setting

From a review of the literature on leadership in priority setting, Reeleder et al (2006, pp 24–5) conclude:

> there is scant empirical data describing the contributions of leadership to priority setting.... A clearer understanding of how priority setting in health services could be improved through effective leadership therefore has not been realised.

Indeed, there is very little in the literature that directly deals with the issue of leadership in priority setting. In an attempt to start to address this gap, Reeleder et al (2006) interviewed chief executive officers of Canadian hospitals to identify their experiences and perceptions of leadership in priority setting (see Table 7.2). Findings suggest the continued importance of factors such as: using evidence; focusing on social values; establishing processes and so on. However, they also highlight the need to develop other skills and carry out other tasks, such as: creating and maintaining relationships; managing networks; delegating; and involving multiple stakeholders.

Table 7.2: Leadership of priority-setting practice and benefits

Domain	Leadership practices for priority setting	Benefits
Foster vision	– Determine vision – Apply strategic planning – Use change management strategies, education and communications – Do not lose sight of long-term time horizon – Focus on core programmes – Emphasise alignment – Focus on key values	– Mobilises stakeholders in common direction – Creates meaning – Enhances feasibility – Creates alignment – Improves services – Improves efficiencies
Create alignment	– Develop shared institutional understanding of vision, values and roles – Ensure 'power triangle' in balance – Align stakeholders – Engage private sector and governments – Collaborate in networks – Manage networks – Establish trust	– Enhances affordability – Enhances fairness – Facilitates service integration – Improves 'buy-in' – Shares resources – Creates innovation – Social capital – Retains autonomy
Develop relationships	– Physician: involve in decision-making – Physician: establish teams – Board: provide context, choices and processes – Staff: delegation – Staff: create trusting milieu – Funder: programme advocacy	– Enhances services to serve public – Provides balance perspectives – Enhances inclusivity – Increases organisational performance – Avoids staff 'push back' – Increases revenues

(continued)

Table 7.2: Leadership of priority-setting practice and benefits (*continued*)

Domain	Leadership practices for priority setting	Benefits
Live values	– Transparency: reveal agendas – Evidence: use criteria and relevant information – Inclusivity: involve relevant stakeholders – Trust: establish trust in relationships – Honesty: manifest honesty in priority setting	– Fairness – Self-evaluation – Cooperation – Affordability – Social capital – Good conduct – Virtue
Establish process	– Promote vision, values and criteria – Enhance planning – Engage stakeholders – Align programmes – Enhance communications – Use challenging goals – Measure progress – Apply clinical programme management – Frame choices – Clarify leadership style	– Fairness – Consensus – Performance – Shared direction – Quality – Alignment – Accountability

Source: Reeleder et al (2006, p 28).

While a minority of the tasks identified relate to the decision-making component of priority setting – such as establishing processes and drawing on evidence – the majority have wider implications, for example, fostering vision, creating alignment and developing relationships. These insights resonate with the broader literature on leadership styles required in complex systems and when tackling wicked problems. In the next sections, therefore, we draw on selected themes from the broader literature in order to suggest strategies for effective leadership in priority setting. In particular, we focus on:

- relational leadership approaches;
- leadership in response to wicked problems; and
- leadership with political awareness.

Relational leadership

Priority setting is often conducted within health care systems that are both complex and rapidly changing. What are required, therefore, are not individual heroic leaders who direct in a one-way fashion, but leadership practices embedded in a system of interdependencies at different levels within organisations. From this perspective, leadership is a relational process, a shared and distributive function dependent on social interactions and networks of influence.

These themes echo the views of priority-setting leaders interviewed by Reeleder et al (2006) who emphasised the importance of relationship-based leadership styles over hierarchical and/or authoritative approaches. For example, due to the complexity of organisational governance and accountability arrangements in health care systems, those leading local processes may not be able to call on sufficient formal authority to mandate the implementation of each of their determinations. In this context, leaders are required to use strategies based on persuasion, facilitation and mediation in order to create a consensus around the need for change. A further implication of the relational model of leadership is that we cannot rely solely on individuals to lead these types of processes and make these effective. The leadership practices identified by Reeleder et al (2006) reflect notions of leadership as a complex adaptive exercise and, therefore, the importance of developing multiple leaders (or 'champions') in priority-setting processes.

The role of the clinical champion is important in this context, as is the relationship between clinical opinion and priority setting more generally. It has been noted that all clinical diagnoses and referrals are resource allocation decisions (Sabin, 1998) and that, therefore, these should be informed by the principle of 'resource stewardship'. There are a number of reasons why more active engagement of the clinical community in priority setting might also be beneficial:

- *Instrumental benefits*: clinical expertise can be invaluable in a decision-making context, especially where the published evidence base is limited and/or inconclusive. In particular, clinicians will have useful knowledge to feed into health profiling of local populations and services affected by resource allocation decisions.
- *Implementation benefits*: lack of coordination between management and clinical functions has long been seen as detrimental to the organisation and delivery of health care (Ham and Dickinson, 2008). Similarly, within the area of priority setting, there is a requirement for clinical buy-in especially in order to ensure the implementation of decisions.
- *Legitimacy benefits*: priority-setting managers invariably call on a smaller pool of public trust than is available to front-line practitioners such as doctors and nurses. These legitimacy deficits can be reduced in situations where clinical champions are involved in making the case both for the need for priority setting in general, and the implementation of specific rationing decisions.
- *Commissioning benefits*: in an English context, the government White Paper *Equity and Excellence* (Secretary of State for Health, 2010) places responsibility for commissioning with GP consortia. This means that plans for allocation of scarce health care resources will need to be adopted and enacted by teams led by clinicians.

However, in order for clinicians to perform a full role in explicit priority setting, resolution of the disjuncture between two perspectives on research is required. Whereas population-based research disciplines inhabit the probabilistic epistemology of techniques such as Health Technology Assessment (HTA) and programme budgeting and marginal analysis (PBMA), clinicians are more inclined to adopt what has been referred to as traditional, deterministic reasoning (Tannenbaum, 1994). This can lead to a 'power struggle' between clinicians and those advocating population-based disciplines such as epidemiology, statistics and health economics (Hunter, 1997). The latter act as 'generic rationalists' seeking to apply standardised decision processes and principles across clinical areas in the pursuit of consistency. By contrast, clinicians traditionally operate more as 'contextual rationalists', mobilising specific sub-areas of expertise and identifying mitigating circumstances and practices to counter unwelcome analysis (Tenbensel, 2002).

Leadership and 'wicked' problems

In Chapter Six, we identified high levels of ambiguity and conflict as key reasons why priority setters often struggle to fully implement rationing decisions. The distinction between decisions that can be implemented in a linear, administrative fashion and those marked by resistance and conflict recalls the distinction in the leadership literature between wicked and tame problems (Grint, 2000). Whilst tame problems require managerial responses, wicked ones require a specific brand of leadership. Also, as with Matland's (1995) matrix, diagnosis of the type of problem has implications for the nature of the power (hard or soft) that can be exercised. Grint summarises the possible scenarios as follows:

• *Critical problems* require an immediate intervention with hard power and therefore demand a command response (where the priority is to provide an answer).
• *Tame problems* are ones that organisations have seen before and thus have an established reaction and require a managerial response (where the priority is to organise a process).
• *Wicked problems* are pernicious social problems where the solution is unclear and require a leadership response that deploys soft power (where the priority is to ask questions).

Table 7.3 lists the potential barriers faced by priority setters and indicates whether these barriers present tame or wicked problems, and, therefore, whether responses require technical or adaptive skills (or a combination of both).

Arguably, one of the most fundamental limitations to current prescriptions for priority setting is the tendency to frame the problem of resource scarcity as tame, and therefore as suited to technical (or managerial) solutions. In practice, technical solutions have foundered on the politically charged, institutionally complex and socially divisive realities of resource allocation in health care. The alternative is to understand and to frame resource scarcity as a wicked issue. Local leaders can therefore play an important role not just in *responding* to the wicked problem of resource scarcity, but also in its construction as a wicked problem in the first place. Successfully framing problems in this way helps to establish the legitimacy and authority required to respond in appropriate ways. What counts as legitimate authority within a situation, therefore, depends on rendering a context persuasively

Table 7.3: Categorising barriers to priority setting

Barrier	Nature of problem	Required response
Lack of evidence	Tame	Technical
Lack of data interpretation skills	Tame	Technical
Inadequate outcome measures	Tame	Technical
Unclear decision processes and criteria	Tame and wicked	Technical and adaptive
Lack of patient and public engagement	Tame and wicked	Technical and adaptive
Complexity of implementation of decisions	Tame and wicked	Technical and adaptive
Lack of awareness from key stakeholders	Tame and wicked	Technical and adaptive
Multiple objectives and values	Wicked	Adaptive
Lack of support from key stakeholders	Wicked	Adaptive
Unrealistic stakeholder expectations	Wicked	Adaptive

and then displaying the appropriate authority style:

> [I]n other words, success is rooted in persuading followers that the problematic situation is either one of a Critical, Tame or Wicked nature and that therefore the appropriate authority form is Command, Management or Leadership in which the role of the decision-maker is to provide the answer, or organize the process or ask the question, respectively. (Grint, 2005a, p 1477)

Drawing on Etzioni's (1964) typology of compliance, Grint argues that the construction of problems and the types of legitimate power and leadership styles may be thought of as set out in Table 7.4. Where problems are *wicked*, we must *lead*; where they are *tame*, we must *manage*; and where they are *critical*, we must *command*. If we believe that a situation is socially constructed and has symbolic resonance, we need to think about what resources are available, what might work best and how to persuade an audience of the validity of our preferred approach. So, where resources might work best in terms of Leadership, the problem should be constructed as wicked. Where Management seems sensible, the problem should be constructed as tame and so on (Grint, 2005a, p 1477).

A key strategy for achieving this is *sensemaking*. If leadership is innately wrapped up in identities and beliefs, it cannot be reduced to individuals simply deploying formal power over others. Rather, in order to persuade multiple stakeholders

Table 7.4: Grint's construction of problems and power

Type of problem	Critical/crisis	Tame	Wicked
Form of authority (legitimate power)	Coercive	Calculative	Normative
Leadership style	Command	Management	Leadership

of the value and legitimacy of priority setting, the leader is required to engage in sensemaking activities. Weick (1995, p 7) argues that 'sensemaking is about authoring as well as reading'; for him, it involves creation as much as discovery. By framing issues in a particular way, sensemaking may be used by leaders to engage members of the group in priority setting. Further, as we have already suggested, leaders might frame issues in certain ways so that they might gain the legitimacy to act in a particular manner. The role of sensemaking is central in actively constructing understandings of concepts and events within the context of health care resource allocation.

The basic proposition that health care resources are scarce and need to be rationed is still rejected by many health care stakeholders and interest groups. However, the experience of many budget-holders is that the gap between demand and supply is widening. Therefore, unless there is wider recognition of the 'problem' that priority setting is designed to address, local processes will not be considered legitimate. The first objective of the priority-setting leader is, therefore, likely to be the *consensual construction of the nature of the problem that priority setting is intended to address*. This will help to create a platform of support for the exploration and implementation of options for addressing this problem – that is, for the priority-setting enterprise itself. This proposition recalls Smircich and Morgan's (1982) argument that acts of leadership only become 'real' in the process of framing and defining reality for followers. At most, therefore, Leaders are the primary symbolising agents within organisations or groups (Bennis, 1994), or, at least, leaders and followers are co-authors (Fairhurst, 1993; Fairhurst and Chandler, 1989; Shotter, 1999).

Leadership with political awareness

A final area of the wider leadership literature that we suggest is important for priority setting is the notion of 'leadership with political awareness' (also known as leadership with political nous or political savvy). A number of the factors that Reeleder et al (2006) identified as being important in leading priority setting can be linked to the notion of leading with political awareness. As noted in the previous chapter, priority setters need to be able to engage with a range of institutions and stakeholders who often have different cultures, values and beliefs. As Hartley notes:

> Many managers have to work with stakeholders who advocate or lobby on behalf of consumer, pressure and political groups ... A globalising world creates a range of uncertainties about world governance, national stability or local priorities which managers need to understand and take account of, and which may have unexpected or substantial repercussions which have to be addressed. (Hartley et al, 2007, p 6)

Douglas and Ammeter (2004, p 537) stress that 'social and political skills are vital to managerial success' and yet research has shown that NHS managers often struggle with aspects of politics and political astuteness. As Hartley and Branicki (2006) argue, this is because there are a number of misconceptions about what political nous is. From a review of the literature these academics argue that politics is often misconstrued in the following ways:

- Politics is the pursuit of self-interest ('politicking') – politics is often seen as being unfair and having no place in rational management systems. This is often associated with the self-interested behaviour of people trying to further their own career.
- Politics is a means to gain market share – this is a 'turf war' and is pursued covertly to win power (Hartley and Branicki, 2006, pp 6–7).

However, there are other understandings of politics that are less negative:

- Politics as a public mechanism for the distribution of resources – politics is an interaction that covers the formal and informal and involves all notions of negotiation and cooperation over the use and distribution of resources.
- Politics as a way of pursuing common purposes and reconciling differences – politics is a constructive means of mobilising support for particular actions by reconciling different interests and values.
- Politics to align individual and organisational objectives – this is about building consensus and reaching beyond difference to coordinate around wider goals despite differences (Hartley and Branicki, 2006, pp 6–7).

These less negative understandings of politics and political astuteness clearly have implications for those who are involved in managing priority setting. If we accept that priority setting is a wicked problem and that local processes are subject to a number of outside influences, we suggest the need for local leaders to develop and exercise political skills and acumen. According to Hartley et al (2007) such skills include:

- shaping key priorities within the organisation;
- building partnerships with external partners;
- promoting the reputation of the organisation; and
- managing risk for the organisation.

Priority-setting leaders, therefore, need to not only gain legitimacy *within* the organisational context, but also amongst external partners and wider civil society. Thus, priority setters cannot just make internally acceptable decisions without due consideration of the broader institutional, political and social settings. In other words, priority setting (and those responsible for leading priority-setting processes) must become attuned to and skilled in the deeper moral and wider political dimensions of health care decision-making. Hartley et al (2007) develop a framework for leading with political astuteness that encapsulates a number of the issues that are raised by Moore's analysis, and which may be helpful in thinking about leadership skills for priority setting (see Box 7.1). As the creators of this framework acknowledge, these types of skills are not entirely distinct from more traditional models of leadership, but the focus on personal integrity and interpersonal skills to provide a solid bedrock for the other dimensions is crucial. These different dimensions are interconnected and, broadly speaking, we might think of these operating at a micro to macro level, with skills 1 and 2 at a more individualistic level than skills 4 and 5.

Box 7.1: Political skills framework

- *Personal skills* – individuals needs to be proactive, self-aware of their motives and behaviours and able to exercise self-control. Individuals must be open to the views of others and initiate actions rather than waiting for things to happen. Personal integrity is crucial to the actions of political leaders.

- *Interpersonal skills* – individuals need to be able to influence the thinking and behaviour of others, particularly gaining buy-in from those that the person has no direct control over. These do not just involve 'soft' skills, but also 'tough' ones as well. Leaders need to be able to handle conflict as well as coaching and mentoring individuals to develop their own political sensitivities and skills further.

- *Reading people and situations* – this is an analytical function and involves understanding the standpoints and values of a range of different stakeholders. It requires thinking about these positions in advance and then dealing with these by drawing on wider knowledge of institutions and social systems to think about what might happen. This is the facet that deals with power and interest groups and their roles within debates.

- *Building alignment and alliances* – this is a crucial skill in terms of action. This concerns how leaders build alliances between stakeholders who might have a wide range of different values and aims. This involves having tough negotiation skills and being able to bring differences out into the open and then being able to deal with these and negotiate these in practice.

- *Strategic direction and scanning* – this relates to purpose and thinking through which issues are important in terms of the future and also how these might impact in practice. So this is more than just horizon scanning and is related to scenario planning and thinking through all the possible options with any one scenario.

Source: Hartley et al (2007, pp 28–30).

Alimo-Metcalfe and Alban–Metcalfe (2005) undertook research to ascertain what effective leadership looks like within a public-sector setting and found some variations in the typical skill set of health care respondents. Although these latter scored highly on measures of decisiveness, they performed less well on accessibility and ability to resolve complex problems. Other relative weaknesses include dimensions that are vital to achieving change in public services, such as:

encouraging the questioning of traditional ways of working; thinking of ways of improving the organisation and the services delivered; and seeking new ways of problem solving. This raises the possibility that many of the functions that appear most important in the leadership of priority setting are currently not effectively carried out. As well as taking responsibility for the formal and structural dimensions of priority setting, we therefore suggest that those in leadership roles also need to consider the strategies set out in Box 7.2.

Box 7.2: Leadership strategies that priority setters should take into consideration

Adopt a relational approach to leading

If, as argued in Chapter Six, priority-setting decisions are only worthwhile when implemented, it is imperative that the leadership role extends to this phase of the process. However, implementation of priority setting takes places in networks as much as it does through hierarchies. Therefore, leadership strategies should reflect the complexity of organisational governance and accountability arrangements in health care systems. In this context, leaders are required to use strategies based on persuasion, facilitation and mediation in order to create a consensus around the need for change.

Tackle priority setting as a 'wicked issue'

Priority setting is often treated as a tame problem that can be overcome using management approaches supported by evidence. However, the majority of priority-setting scenarios and features conform to the notion of wicked issues in the sense that there are high levels of ambiguity and conflict and long-standing, intractable barriers to implementation.

Encourage sensemaking

If, as argued again in Chapter Six, legitimacy and support for priority setting are as important as making the correct priority-setting decisions, then sensemaking is likely to be a key component of the leadership role. In particular, this will require the development of a broad consensus around the need to ration care. Sensemaking will also be required when tackling the complex and highly charged business of removing or withholding services.

Develop political acumen

An explicitly politically adept approach to leadership focuses on the need to understand the macro-political (ie governmental) influences on decisions and their implementation as well as drawing attention to the importance of building alliances and protecting local processes against unreasonable attack from disaffected interest groups.

Chapter summary

Although leadership is often cited as an important component of priority setting, there is, as yet, little written about this topic. Priority setting is frequently treated as a tame problem and, therefore, subject to technical, management solutions. In this chapter, we have argued for its reframing as a wicked issue, which requires leadership, and Reeleder et al's (2006) description of leadership activity in priority setting appears to support this claim. Important considerations are, therefore, the need for relational leadership styles, engaging in sensemaking and developing political savvy. However, these are skills and orientations that are not necessarily embedded in current health care management roles, and we must avoid naive assumptions as to the extent of autonomy afforded to leaders of local processes. In other words, if explicit priority setting is to be granted the status of a legitimate management practice, leaders will require support. The extent to which they can engender this support by adopting the strategies outlined in this chapter remains open to question as this is an area that requires much more research, debate and exploration than is currently available within the priority-setting literature.

EIGHT

Disinvestment as a priority-setting case study

Key points covered in Chapter Eight

- Disinvestment is especially important in times of economic deficit.
- Priority setting has tended to focus on allocation of additional resources and has therefore neglected the issue of allocating dwindling budgets.
- Health Technology Assessment (HTA) and programme budgeting and marginal analysis (PBMA) are examples of important tools for deciding which interventions and services should be disinvested in.
- Legitimacy, accountability and implementation barriers are heightened when priority setters seek to withdraw or reduce services.
- The range of strategies available to priority setters – as well as leadership skills – needs to be employed in the disinvestment process.

Introduction

As noted in Chapter One, disinvestment is important when budgets are either frozen or subject to cuts. This can take a number of forms. One option is the removal from the 'list' of approved interventions on grounds of opportunity cost (in much the same way as lists of decommissioned practices are compiled on grounds of adverse effects). In other words, treatments would be decommissioned that are deemed to be an inefficient use of public resources. However, other forms of disinvestment may include retraction (investing in less of an intervention), restriction (withdrawing treatment from patient subgroups) and substitution (replacing a practice with one deemed more efficient). The objectives of disinvestment can also vary; for example, from a concern to reduce overall spend to an emphasis on reallocation of savings to more beneficial areas of service. Like all rationing, disinvestment can be carried out in an implicit manner (whereby old practices die a slow death rather than being decommissioned), although the concern here is with the adoption of explicit approaches.

In whatever form, at the current time there is an urgent need for the nettle of disinvestment to be grasped. However, the challenges resource allocators face are heightened when priority setting is applied to the question of withdrawal of health care services. This chapter uses the topic of disinvestment to crystallise many of the arguments presented throughout the text – notably, the need to address issues of ethics, involvement, accountability, legitimacy and implementation – while also offering specific insights into an increasingly important area of health system policy and activity. It begins with a summary of current strategies for generating a disinvestment evidence base before considering management techniques such as PBMA. Finally, recent research carried out by the authors is drawn upon in a discussion of the barriers to the implementation of disinvestment, and strategies for overcoming these.

Prescriptions for disinvestment

Health Technology Assessment

The rate of development of expensive new health care interventions is one of the key drivers of resource scarcity. In England and Wales, NICE's technology appraisal programme has expanded in response to the need for evidence reviews of these new technologies. However, local decision-makers remain inundated with requests for technologies for which no central guidance exists. Furthermore, many services that were implemented before cost-effectiveness became a common criterion of treatment coverage remain in place, a situation that has been characterised as being 'stuck with the old and overwhelmed by the new' (Elshaug et al, 2007, p 25). NICE currently approves new technologies if they bring about extra clinical benefit at an acceptable additional cost (the much discussed 'cost-effectiveness threshold'). It has, however, been criticised for not balancing its budget-inflating advice with equivalent recommendations for making savings (Gallego et al, 2010). The Institute has recognised the validity of these criticisms and declared an intention to 'purge from the NHS treatments that do not improve health or are poor value for money' (Kmietowicz, 2006, p 568) by compiling a 'do not do' interventions database (see www.nice.org.uk/usingguidance/donotdorecommendations/index.jsp). Selecting health care practices as candidates for disinvestment clearly requires comparative research and review; however, this evidence base is currently underdeveloped (Ibargoyen-Roteta et al, 2009), and attention has therefore focused on filling the data gap. Elshaug et al (2009) postulate criteria for both the identification of candidates for disinvestment, and further selection of those to be subject to detailed review (see Box 8.1).

Box 8.1: Criteria for selecting candidates for disinvestment

a) Criteria for short-listing candidates for assessment
  – New evidence suggests review required
  – Variations in clinical practice suggest differing views of an interventions value
  – Practices appear inconsistent with clinical guidelines
  – The technology has changed/development since the time of its implementation
  – Public, clinical and professional opinion suggests that an intervention should be assessed
  – A formal nomination process identifies a technology as a candidate for assessment
  – A new intervention appears to duplicate an existing practice

b) Criteria for identifying candidates for detailed review
  – Cost of the intervention
  – Outcomes and impact of the intervention (and relevance of these)
  – Costs and outcomes of alternatives
  – Disease burden
  – Strength of evidence (and scope for evidence generation)

Source: Adapted from Elshaug et al (2009).

As useful as these criteria are, they require validation as acceptable grounds for withdrawing health care practices. In other words, as with all priority setting, disinvestment decision criteria need to reflect the value-based preferences of citizens, as derived from deliberative exercises described in Chapter Three (as well as through macro-political, democratic processes). Obtaining the necessary evidence to inform analysis can pose additional problems with the disinvestment evidence base very much in its infancy – not just in terms of comparative assessment, but also with respect to the costs to, and impact upon, local systems. The limits of HTA methods are identified in a UK Treasury report (cited in Elshaug et al, 2007) in which it is stated:

> The delivery of robust scientific appraisal for technologies is coming under increasing challenge as a result of its reliance on methodologies that, it is widely recognised, need further development, given that Health Technology Assessment (HTA) is a relatively new science. Appropriate research is required to address these challenges. In particular, research into methodologies for ... disinvestment methods. (Cooksey, 2006, p 23)

The absence of consensus on criteria for disinvestment combined with weaknesses in the evidence base again point to the need for robust decision-making *processes*, such as those introduced in Chapter Two. Arguably, the need for decision processes to be robust to challenge is greater when the primary objective is disinvestment.

Programme budgeting and marginal analysis

Each of the tools included in multi-criteria approaches introduced in Chapter Five are capable of being adapted to assist with disinvestment. For example, programme budgeting (PB) has been advocated as a tool for identifying areas to reduce spending (Nuti et al, 2010). PBMA is discussed here as an example of a management tool that has been advanced as a solution to the problems posed by the need to disinvest (Donaldson et al, 2010). This framework (described in detail in Chapter Five) is one of a number in existence that aim to apply the principles of opportunity cost and the margin to management decision-making in the area of resource allocation. PBMA is more practical than an HTA-led approach as it relies less on access to perfect data, instead adopting a pragmatic approach that combines formal evidence with local data and expert opinion to determine the likely costs and outcomes of options for investment of resources. The involvement of local stakeholders means that there is flexibility in identifying measures of cost and outcomes that are relevant to context (rather than insisting on generalised summary measures such as the Quality-Adjusted Life Year) and in applying these measures to a range of programme decisions. Advocates have asserted PBMA to be the only form of 'rational disinvestment' available to local decision-makers and one that promises to most fairly distribute the harms that accompany overall reductions in health care investment (Donaldson et al, 2010). PBMA also combines elements of pluralism when informed by substantial decision conferencing and deliberation between stakeholders.

However, there are limitations to the PBMA approach, especially when applied to disinvestment. As a costly and time-consuming exercise, there needs to be an incentive for local (especially clinical) involvement. Clearly, exhortation (ie emphasising the importance of taking a balanced approach to cutting spending) will be effective for some, but others may require more convincing of the value of sacrificing their time. Also, whereas a PBMA approach to the allocation of *additional* resources may have positive appeal to local service providers, an agenda of *disinvestment* may not. In a similar vein, it has been noted that candidates for extra investment tend to be more readily identified than candidates for disinvestment (Gallego et al, 2010). These concerns suggest the need for careful consideration of how the PBMA disinvestment process is to be incentivised.

The material introduced in Chapters Six and Seven raised questions over the ease with which priority-setting decisions can be implemented in difficult political climates and complex systems. These concerns are no less apposite in relation to disinvestment. Gallego et al (2010, p 8) note the resistance of stakeholder groups to the withdrawal of services:

> As disinvestment will create losses, to clinicians, to consumers and to providers of the technology, there will be strong resistance to any active withdrawal of funding. At the same time, the additional benefits

and/or savings from any disinvestments may not be realised for a considerable period of time.

Disinvestment is a 'hard sell' and runs the risk of sabotage by the powerful interest groups affected. In this context, implementation tools such as clinical guidelines are likely to be a necessary but insufficient tool for changing the behaviour of professionals and organisations resistant to the proposed removal of a treatment. The next section illustrates the implementation difficulties that can arise when priority setters seek to advance a disinvestment agenda.

The implementation gap

NHS Morebeck

Recent research by the authors has investigated priority setting in English Primary Care Trusts (PCTs) (Robinson et al, 2011b). A major theme of the study was the economic crisis and the financial pressures that this presaged for local budget-holders. Data from one of the case studies is presented here as an illustration of the implementation barriers faced by local decision-makers and how these are exacerbated when attempting disinvestment. 'NHS Morebeck' had established a board with responsibility for reviewing and planning the entire spend of the PCT. This in itself represented a step forward from the more typical approach to priority setting in which models are applied only to additional monies as these become available. Furthermore, NHS Morebeck had secured buy-in and representation from a wide range of agencies operating in the local area including: all relevant PCT departments; local government; managers of relevant provider organisations (including the local acute hospitals); and clinicians from across primary and secondary care.

The board had also taken a proactive, evidence-based approach to the identification of options for investment and disinvestment, primarily in the form of an externally commissioned PBMA exercise that had resulted in identification of eight technologies and services for investment and disinvestment. This was the first time that participants could recall there being such cross-locality commitment to shared decision-making and for independently conducted analysis to have fed into this. At the time of data collection, the board had met on a number of occasions to oversee implementation, within the local delivery system, of the determinations reached:

Interviews with participants suggested that early enthusiasm had become tempered with frustration at the lack of progress in implementing changes to services:

> "There is lots of time and investment from the senior team but very little return on investment. It's great we are all getting together. The PCT is only 3 years old and individuals from across the health economy have never really come together this way … but we need some wins

otherwise people will lose interest and nothing will be achieved. I do feel frustrated that we have not done more."

"Just getting clinicians involved in discussions is not in itself enough … the work's been really slow and I fear we are really losing engagement because clinicians are coming to meaningless meetings, we are being asked to engage but then nothing happens."

"There are great and grand ideas about service redesign, lots of talking around the edges but no one really discussing how we will make savings. These are difficult financial times so what are we going to stop doing? That is the real question."

"It's a bit of a talking shop."

Respondents were concerned that the momentum of the process had been lost at the implementing phase, and noted a number of possible reasons for this, including divergent organisational strategies, and a lack of governance and performance management mechanisms:

"On the ground, we have a lack of support. The balance is not good. We need project managers holding people to account. It's not good that we have been milling around in this pond forever. I'm not sure we have the correct governance structures in place."

"The real issue which no one wants to discuss is who realises the benefit or loss of a decision…. We just can't seem to have these discussions. We have not got the sophistication and managerial competencies to do this and to work out how to make changes to the money flow. It feels like we are in a tanker and we can't move the money around."

These barriers were most formidable in the area of disinvestment where divisions between organisations involved in the process were most likely to emerge:

"Disinvestment is not easy because that could be a big chunk of our income being removed. But if we are going to have proper transformation, then we need to make sure we can deliver on that. It's a balancing act, but we need to look at things as a health economy rather than having organisational boundaries. Egos get in the way. The focus is on my organisation rather than a shared approach. If you were an alien landing from mars you would never understand that the NHS was one organisation."

The political fallout of rationing was also seen as extending to the broader public, for whom disinvestment was considered unacceptable. Interestingly, those designing the priority-setting process had decided that public involvement was not required in the process of identification of services for disinvestment:

> "There are both organisational and professional barriers ... oh and the public – you try and close an [accident and emergency] department or close a hospital. It just creates such a political atmosphere. I think something needs to happen nationally. I think the NHS is too fat and there are some things we need to take locally, but there needs to be some fairly big national positions on stuff. Locally, we need discussions on professional and organisational self interest. Someone needs to be seen to be taking the lead and having those discussions."

This comment was typical of a broader concern that the difficult business of disinvestment could not be led entirely by local commissioners and that there was a need for government involvement and support. However, the overall political context was experienced as unhelpful, especially inasmuch as it militated against the kinds of rational planning required:

> "The NHS is really unstable. There is constant pressure to do things quickly, meet targets, save money and, on the other hand, we don't take time to look at what is stable, we don't really know where we are going. It's just constant reaction, no planning."

These comments proved somewhat prophetic. Within months, a new government had announced plans for a reorganisation of the NHS, including the abolishment of PCT commissioning (Secretary of State for Health, 2010). The 'implementation gap' of priority setting (and disinvestment) was therefore attributed to a number of factors, including:

• a lack of relevant information and evidence on the implementation process;
• a lack of project management support for the implementation of priority-setting decisions;
• governance structures that were inadequate for ensuring delivery of priority-setting decisions;
• a general lack of linkage between the decision-making function and the wider health care delivery system;
• organisational and professional resistance;
• hostility to disinvestment from the public and media; and
• a lack of clear political support and direction.

Chapter summary

Disinvestment is important to health care systems and this is especially so within a context of overall budget reductions. Improving HTA and adopting management techniques such as PBMA are important in making disinvestment decisions, as is the adoption of process-based criteria and carrying out meaningful public participation exercises. The case study of NHS Morebeck reinforces some of the key messages of the book so far. In particular, it suggests that progress in reaching decisions is only half of the priority-setting process, and that issues of governance, institutions, legitimacy and power remain crucial in successful delivery against these agreed priorities (Robinson et al, 2011a). The persistence of a low-profile, 'closed session' approach to decision-making also seems at odds with the need to create a coalition of support for the rationing enterprise.

Importantly, the study also suggests that failure to implement disinvestment is not necessarily 'irrational' and might instead be understood as a logical consequence of the political and institutional arrangements within which decision-makers operate. This has profound implications for those seeking to make recommendations to such bodies. In this context, the further production of decision evidence and analysis would be largely redundant and cannot be seen as a suitable response to the difficulties faced. Instead, prescriptions would be more usefully focused on reviewing basic functions and responsibilities as well as addressing an unreceptive climate for the entire rationing enterprise. Cast as a programme of change, disinvestment processes will require skilled expertise in change management and a shared commitment to implementation. This was articulated in a recent *British Medical Journal* editorial where it was observed: 'We lack a shared common language, a vocabulary, and a narrative of change for discussing the subject. Without this an integrated policy of disinvestment will be difficult to introduce' (Cooper and Starkey, 2010, p 605). The need to construct a 'common language' and a 'narrative for change' highlights the relational, adaptive and political dimensions of the leadership of disinvestment.

Overall, disinvestment (in its various forms) presents considerable challenges, including: the need to establish agreement over the criteria by which decisions will be taken; the need to develop a thorough understanding of the full range of current services and areas of investment and their performance against these criteria; the need to manage and negotiate the political hazards and fallout associated with the removal/withdrawal of services; and the difficulty of implementing substitution and disinvestment in complex systems. In order to make efficiency savings and to release funds, tough choices will need to be made, and there will inevitably be losers as a result. This in itself necessitates a culture shift for many health care institutions. Such a change requires a combination of leadership, strategic goals, technical capacity and information resources. It will also need broad public support at both the national and local level, with large-scale public engagement over the aims and means of health care.

NINE

Conclusions

Introduction

Resource scarcity in health care can be seen as both a tame and wicked issue. It is 'tame' in the sense that it is not new, and there are strategies available to help combat its consequences. For example, most governments have introduced cost-containment measures designed to curtail the rise in health care expenditure, including setting budget ceilings on acute and other provider organisations. This has meant that many of the difficult decisions regarding the distribution of scarce resources have often been made in a low-profile or opaque manner, by clinicians and others working at ground level. Some commentators argue that this remains the most efficacious approach to rationing, and that explicit approaches are too damaging to public and patient trust in services (Mechanic, 1995).

However, implicit rationing carries its own risks and pitfalls and is increasingly agreed to be ethically and politically unacceptable (Sulmasy, 1992). This text has therefore proceeded from the assumption that explicit priority setting is a legitimate and necessary feature of contemporary policy and practice in health care. But priority setting falls within the category of those policy problems deemed 'wicked'. This is because simple solutions have proved elusive for reasons that go beyond a shortage of effective management tools. We believe that the literature on priority setting contains much that is valuable and, indeed, essential to effective practice. The first half of this text has therefore been dedicated to explaining and critiquing developments in areas of: ethics, processes, involvement, evidence and analysis. However, in recognition of the limits to strategies that portray priority setting as tame, we have also explored the barriers and facilitators relating to politics, institutions and perception, and the types of leadership responses that these factors demand. This chapter brings together each of these themes and summarises the key messages for those responsible for health care priority setting and resource allocation.

Beyond rationalism versus pluralism

We noted in the introduction that much of the priority-setting literature is marked by a polarisation between advocates of two distinct forms of 'rationality'. On one side is the instrumentalism of the rational model, which advocates rules-based priority setting towards *optimal* decision outcomes. On the other side sit exponents of debate, involvement and consensus-building in the pursuit of *satisfactory* or acceptable decision outcomes. Key areas of dispute include the relative emphasis on: principles and process; evidence and debate; and information and institutions. In this section, we attempt a reconciliation and development of these positions in the light of the themes presented thus far.

Many commentators believe that priority setting should follow accepted and agreed principles. For example, traditional health economics has taken it as a first principle that scarce resources should be allocated so as to maximise population health, possibly with some adjustment for equity concerns (Williams, 1997). However, advocacy of population health maximisation has been shown to exclude other principles that may be of importance to the public. These include the 'rule of rescue' (whereby life-saving interventions are seen as paramount) and respect for individual human dignity (Hadorn, 1991a; Jagsi et al, 2004). To these can be added the values of equity and distributive justice, as well as the 'precepts of access and treatment on which the NHS is founded' (Syrett, 2003, p 742). Definitively held public values are therefore hard to pin down and societies have become sufficiently diverse for some commentators to posit an 'irreducible pluralism' preventing attainment of a unified normative stance (Schlander, 2008, p 535) and the need, therefore, to shift attention to the *processes* by which rationing decisions are made. For example, Daniels (2000, p 1301) argues:

> In pluralist societies we are likely to find reasonable disagreement about principles that should govern priority setting. For example, some will want to give more priority to the worst off, some less; some will be willing to aggregate benefits in ways that others are not. In the absence of consensus on principles, a fair process allows us to agree on what is legitimate and fair.

Clearly, the establishment of sound decision-making processes does not exclude attempts to identify underlying ethical principles and vice versa. However, while work to better understand the rationing values of the public is ongoing (eg Cookson and Dolan, 2000), the pursuit of participative decision-making models remains important.

A second tension concerns the role that evidence and expertise play and should play in the decision-making process. The assumption that increasing and improving the evidence base of decisions will bring about corresponding rationalisation of the decision-making processes, and its outputs, is at the heart of the evidence-based approach, and since the 1990s there has been an explosion in the use of Health Technology Assessment (HTA) within OECD countries. However, the rise of HTA does not appear to have brought about a depoliticisation of priority setting and technocratic approaches have not always delivered the expected reductions in overall spend (Ham and Coulter, 2001). Furthermore, there is a dearth of evidence to support disinvestment in the broader sweep of existing practices that may or may not be an effective use of NHS resources. Critics have argued that rationalist, technocratic approaches attempt to erase fundamental questions of value from the prioritisation process (Gelijns et al, 2005) and instead advocate a systematic policy of public involvement in the prioritisation process, focusing on the need for consensus and deliberation (eg Sackett et al, 1997; Harrison, 1998; Robinson, 1999).

These debates suggest that there are currently weaknesses in both the information available for priority setting and the institutional capacities of bodies charged with decision-making. The optimal allocation of future resources between these two areas is also argued over, most notably in a conference debate between political scientist Rudolph Klein and health economist Alan Williams (Klein and Williams, 2000). In this exchange, Williams advocates a focus on information-based solutions to the pursuit of health service objectives, seeing this as an antidote to structural reorganisations that neither draw upon nor generate useful evidence. However, as Klein sees it, energy would be better spent in improving the health service's decision-making capacity through the development of inclusive institutions:

> The reason why I give primacy to institutions as against information is that unless we strengthen our institutional capacity to analyse evidence, to clarify policy choices and to promote informed debate, generating more information is more likely to compound confusion than to lead to better decision making. (Klein and Williams, 2000, p 24)

The question of balance between information-based approaches and a focus on designing better institutions is a complex one that requires assessment of the extent of polarity (and mutual exclusivity) of the two perspectives presented. A key issue for this book has been the respective importance of information and institutional capacity in priority setting and we argue that the relationship between institutions and information needs to be revisited. The Klein–Williams debate presents a false dichotomy when considered in the light of the complex interaction between structural context and decision-makers' demand for information. For example, when creating NICE (and its technology appraisals programme in particular), the government was at pains to ensure that the experts, researchers and decision-makers involved would be insulated from the tricky business of policy implementation and the attendant requirements for bargaining and mutual adjustment between partisan stakeholders. The logic behind this was that fairness and legitimacy would best be served through the objectivity of an evidence-based approach. In accordance with this, external stakeholders seeking to challenge appraisal determinations are expected to adopt a similar commitment to the tenets of quantitative decision analysis, rather than the more traditional 'special pleading' of winners and losers in the policy process. Under these circumstances, it is no surprise that the decision-making process itself creates a demand for formal evidence. This has proved to be a necessary – if not sufficient – step to the attainment of defendable determinations. In the process, some form of case law, as enshrined in a cost-effectiveness threshold below which all new treatments are recommended, has developed.

Local institutions do not work in the same way. A number of features of the decision-making environment militate against emphasis on evidence and analysis, including: unclear relationships with resource allocators; an explicitly political decision-making process; poorly specified decision-making criteria; and incompatible policy frames. Of far more importance to local resource allocators is the concern to control spending in departments, directorates and organisations, and to satisfy the demands of internal and local interest groups. Correspondingly, both the degree and type of information will differ from national guidance-producing bodies such as NICE. This underlines the assertion that information of any type is generally only considered important when the broader environment creates the demand for it. This is not to suggest that the quality and reliability of information is unimportant or that evidence does not have a role to play in priority setting. It does imply, however, that those who seek to promote the efficient and equitable distribution of scarce resources must avoid naivety. Information is only as influential as politics, institutions and values allow.

The symbiosis of information and institutions is noted by Ham and Robert (2003, p 156) who suggest that 'strengthening the institutional framework for priority setting is likely to increase the demand for and use of information, whether or not this is planned'. We agree and would extend this further: institutional frameworks must also facilitate *implementation* of priority-setting decisions and this will require access to information on impact, performance and outcomes, alongside information to support decisions. The importance of implementation – a recurring theme of this text – is overlooked in much of the existing priority-setting literature, which instead concentrates mainly on decision-making, and then laments the minimal impact of these decisions on actual practice (Sabik and Lie, 2008). A key reason for this disjuncture is the messy realities of resource allocation in complex health care systems. In our view, it is unhelpful and inappropriate to insulate decision-makers from the task of putting into practice recommendations deriving from priority-setting processes. We therefore argue for a decoupling of priority setting and decision-making (the latter is only one element of the former) and for a focus on the challenges of changing practice.

Clearly, this requires us to connect priority setting to the broader literature on change, innovation and improvement in health care (Williams and Dickinson, 2010). However, the highly political and emotive nature of rationing, and the problems of legitimacy that undermine attempts to take an explicit approach to priority setting, require us to look not just inwards at systems and practices, but also upwards towards government and outwards towards civic society as it is in these arenas that the struggle for trust and legitimacy will be played out. Rationing requires forms of leadership that do not shy away from the task of engaging this authorising environment and leaders with political astuteness.

Understanding priority setting

Priority setting is about more than decision processes and outcomes. Table 9.1 attempts to map the layers of priority setting with respect to:

- *Settings* – these refer to the arenas that shape the success or failure of priority setting as an instrument of resource allocation. As well as the decision-making context (which may itself involve a series of points such as public engagement exercises, data collection and analysis, deliberation between participants in priority-setting processes and so on), attention needs to be paid to the settings within which priority setting is implemented, and to broader political and social spheres that ultimately will determine whether the outcomes of decision processes are accepted or rejected.
- *Actors* – involvement in decision-making is likely to take different forms in each of these settings. Although no definitive prescription for when and how to involve different actors in priority setting is offered here, we would suggest that those given formal responsibility for reaching priority-setting determinations cannot do so without substantive and ongoing input from actors located in wider settings. In particular, this includes those responsible for the implementation of decisions and those (government and citizens) with the democratic authority to influence resource allocation priorities. Furthermore, it is unlikely to be sufficient to draft a small number of 'representatives' from these wider spheres into the 'inner circle' of decision-making. This may seem onerous; however, we contend that the benefits (instrumental, political and educative) of genuinely shared decision-making outweigh the extra time and resources this requires.
- *Information* – this refers to the types of evidence, knowledge and analysis required for successful priority setting in each of these respects. Decision analysis of some form is clearly a useful aid to priority setters. However, arguably as important is information on the likely impact on delivery settings. This latter might include: budget impact data; the tacit knowledge of professionals responsible for leading change and implementation; and the insights and experiences of service users implicated in proposed changes to services. Finally, priority setting requires information on the wider contexts. This might include: analysis of the macro-policy climate (ie the priorities and expectations of government in relation to health care) and appreciation of wider socio-cultural mores and how these impact on attitudes towards health.

We therefore propose that priority setting in health care take account of these three contexts when considering who should be involved and what information is made available. Furthermore, we argue that each of the substantive dimensions discussed in this book should be accounted for when designing and implementing

Table 9.1: Priority-setting contexts, actors and analysis

Contexts	Actors	Analysis
Decision-making functions	Decision-makers and citizens	Decision analysis
Implementing systems and networks	Implementers, users and stakeholders	System impact and affordability analysis
Political and social environment	Government and media	Acceptability analysis

priority-setting policies at local levels of health care. These include: goals; processes; engagement; evidence; institutions; politics; and leadership. The relevance of these is briefly reprised in Table 9.2.

Table 9.2: Aspects of priority setting

Element	Relevance to priority setting
Goals	These are the (instrumental) ethical values underpinning priority setting. They are likely to be multiple and, therefore, trade-offs between them will be required.
Processes	Good processes can have intrinsic value (ie in supporting and empowering those involved), but are also central to the delivery of the goals of priority setting. Strong processes are also important to accountability and broader legitimacy.
Engagement	Engagement with stakeholders and the public is a feature of good decision-making processes in terms of achieving high levels of decision quality and appropriateness. It can also have intrinsic value in terms of democratic accountability and education. However, engagement strategies need to be sophisticated and account for power imbalances amongst stakeholder groups and between these and decision-makers.
Evidence	Generating evidence adds value primarily in its contribution to decision quality and appropriateness – for example, enabling analysis of decision options, outcomes and implementation.
Institutions	Organisations and institutions can either help or hinder priority setting. The relationship between the decision-making function and broader resource allocation and decision implementation systems (as well as cultures) is therefore crucial.
Politics	None of the above elements are sufficient to ensure legitimacy for priority setting, although each can play a role in this. If the political environment – made up of, for example, the demands and expectations of government and the attitudes of wider society – is not supportive of the priority-setting process, it is likely to fail, irrespective of its quality and rigour.
Leadership	Priority setting is not a purely technical exercise and can be understood as a response to a series of wicked problems. Like all aspects of public-sector strategy, organisation and delivery, priority setting requires effective management. As an area marked by high levels of dispute, ambiguity and emotion, it also requires effective leadership at multiple levels.

Evaluating priority setting

We propose this list of 'ingredients' as the basis for an evaluative framework, on the grounds that the extent to which these seven dimensions are in place and aligned is likely to determine, in large part, the success or otherwise of priority setting. We therefore add this, as yet under-developed, evaluative framework to that provided by Sibbald et al (2009) who identify 10 aspects of 'successful' priority setting (see Box 9.1). Ultimately, however, methods for review and assessment should reflect evaluation aims (for a more detailed exploration of the options available for evaluation of priority setting, see Smith et al, 2011).

Box 9.1: Understanding 'success' in priority setting

- *Stakeholder engagement* – this includes involvement of administrators, clinicians, members of the public and patients. Engagement should take multiple forms including round tables, open forums, departmental meetings. Engagement requires genuine partnership and empowerment.
- *Stakeholder understanding* – the degree to which stakeholders have gained insight into and understand all aspects of the priority-setting process.
- *Stakeholder acceptance and satisfaction* – as indicated by continued willingness to participate in and support the process.
- *Explicit process* – the extent to which stakeholders know who is making the decision as well as how and why the decision will be made. This requires effective communication via multiple vehicles.
- *Information management* – the extent to which appropriate information is made available to decision-makers during the priority-setting process, and how effectively this information is collected and collated.
- *Consideration of values and context* – this includes values of individuals, organisations and other stakeholders. 'Context' refers to the broader health care environment, strategic directions and so on.
- *Revision or appeals mechanism* – whether the process has a formal mechanism for the review of decisions, and for addressing disagreements constructively.
- *Shifted resources* – the extent to which priority setting results in allocation (and reallocation) of budgets across portfolios and other changes in use of resources and/or strategic directions.
- *Decision-making quality* – the extent to which the following is demonstrated: use of available evidence; consistency of reasoning; institutionalisation of the priority-setting process; alignment with stated goals; adherence to stated process; and ongoing learning and improvement.
- *Positive externalities* – as indicated by: positive media coverage; peer-emulation; and/or health sector recognition.

Source: Adapted from Sibbald et al (2009).

Doing priority setting

Knowing what priority setting involves and actually doing it are, of course, two different things. In this section, we look at implications for the practice of priority setting and draw out a summary of broad recommendations from the more detailed discussions provided throughout this text.

Goals

Priority setting is ultimately judged by the extent to which it reflects the social value preferences of the society that funds and is served by it. Priority setters cannot assume to know what the important principles are as these are not self-evident. It is likely that decisions will have to reflect a trade-off between egalitarian (distributing resources fairly), individualist (recognising the rights of the individual) and utilitarian (maximising benefit) considerations. These are tensions that are played out in government policy and popular discourse in every country of the developed world and in arenas ranging from government to households. Priority setters cannot be expected to resolve these issues by themselves. Rather they should actively engage with, and at times lead, broader discussions over the underlying purposes of health care so that their decisions are informed by an ongoing dialogue with wider society. Practical strategies for tackling issues of value include deliberative engagement with the public and the adoption (and adaption) of ethical frameworks to assess investment and disinvestment options.

Processes

It is now widely accepted that priority setting is about more than getting the 'right' answer. If decisions are not arrived at via a process that is considered open and fair, they will not be accepted as legitimate. Priority setters, therefore, need a plan for how they intend to involve stakeholders and the public. Accountability for reasonableness draws attention to important measures of process in priority setting. Beyond this a number of dimensions should be accounted for, such as how the deliberative component of decision-making proceeds (ie according to what criteria and processes) and the influence of power and framing in this. By setting terms of reference for how these micro-processes will proceed, decision-makers can increase fairness and accountability.

Engagement

This book has argued for the importance of the widespread involvement of stakeholders in priority setting, while cautioning against naive prescriptions for 'getting everyone round the table'. Those designing priority-setting arrangements need to be aware of the extent to which decision-making is structured to encourage bargaining between sectional interest groups – for example, over the financial burden of implementation. Consideration, therefore, needs to be given to questions such as:

• What role are those involved expected to play? For example, how are the dual roles of *expert* (bearers of specialist knowledge on decision content or analysis) and *representative* (those advocating on behalf of interests perceived to be legitimate influencers of decisions) accommodated?

- How will power imbalances be accounted for in the process of involvement? For example, the public invariably exercise less authority than managers and the medical profession and this can skew decision outcomes.
- How will differences of opinion be accommodated and/or resolved?
- How will the views of those engaged be fed into outcomes?

There are no simple answers to these questions. However, they are considerations that should be built into the design and delivery of priority-setting processes, into the terms and references of decision-making bodies, and into the roles and responsibilities designated to those recruited to take part.

Evidence

In this book, we have focused on evidence as provided by techniques such as economic evaluations and multi-criteria decision analysis. However, these may not always be the appropriate or preferred approach. For example, needs analysis will also be important to decisions and cost–impact assessments may be required for implementation of decisions. In terms of capacity for data generation and interpretation, we suggest that the following questions are addressed:

- What data can and should be developed by the decision-makers (eg information on local budgets, local population needs, current service capacity)?
- What evidence is available 'off the shelf' (eg HTAs, economic evaluations)?
- Alternatively, which should be commissioned from outside agencies (eg programme budgeting and marginal analysis, socio-technical approach)?
- What information might be best commissioned in conjunction with other local decision-makers (eg joint health and social care needs analysis, de novo, locally specific economic decision analysis)?
- What internal analytical skills are required to interpret, critique and apply the evidence base?
- What additional analytical expertise should be commissioned as and when required?

In order to be useful, it is necessary that evidence and analysis are seen by end users to be relevant (ie providing data on parameters that are likely to influence the decisions of the policymakers) and appropriate to the decisions they face, taking into account relevant contextual factors (eg budgetary arrangements commonly seen in the NHS), and that such analyses are seen as providing information that can inform the implementation of decisions in a complex environment. Addressing these questions should help to maximise relevance.

Institutions

Those designing priority-setting processes need to give consideration to where these sit in relation to broader structures of accountability, decision-making and implementation. For example, clarification and formalisation of the role of the priority-setting mechanism in the actual allocation of resources is crucial. Questions to consider include:

• Should priority setting be exclusively located in the health care commissioning process?
• If so, what is the formal role of government and/or provider networks in these decisions?
• Should hospitals retain some discretion over entry and exit from formulary lists?
• Should priority-setting decisions be made binding upon all relevant budget-holders and, if so, what is the mechanism for achieving this?

Addressing such questions could start the process of establishing more accountable, consistent and informed priority-setting and resource allocation arrangements. This focus on process, evidence and standardisation in turn offers some defence for embattled and occasionally beleaguered decision-makers subject to accusations of the unfair or unreasonable withholding of treatment. Alignment is also required with respect to incentives and strategic planning. It is not enough for actors to engage in a priority-setting process if they remain bound by separate and competing organisational, strategic priorities. The priority-setting enterprise, therefore, needs to be aligned with the strategic plans and priorities of cooperating and implementing organisations and networks.

Management techniques will also be required to facilitate implementation of priority-setting decisions. For example, these may include:

• process mapping in order to understand and secure agreement on roles and responsibilities in decision implementation;
• employing effective governance regimes to incentivise and facilitate the implementation of priority-setting decisions;
• performance management of delivery against priority-setting decisions; and
• setting up feedback and information loops and overall management of the explicit and tacit knowledge required to make changes to practice required by priority-setting decisions.

Politics

Identifying priorities is a necessary but insufficient part of the resource allocation process. As well as understanding the relationship between priority setting and the institutional constraints in which this operates, there is a requirement for greater clarity with regard to responsibilities within a broader political context.

Moore's concept of the 'authorising environment' is helpful here in directing decision-makers towards the importance of establishing trust and buy-in to the priority-setting enterprise. Questions that those leading prioritisation might usefully ask here include:

- What government frameworks and policies impact on and/or constrain local priority setting?
- What is the nature of the relationship between the priority-setting function and: government agencies; service providers; or key partner agencies?
- What are other important aspects of context that will influence responses to priority-setting models and decisions (eg local history and community)?
- What is the profile of the priority-setting organisation/panel/process within the media and broader public?
- What levels of trust currently exist within and between these parties?

The need to maximise trust ought to be at the heart of attempts to secure support for priority setting. Answers to the above questions should help priority setters target relationships where legitimacy deficits are likely to be most extreme (and therefore most damaging), and to concentrate energies on repairing and/or improving these.

Leadership and management

We would argue that making best use of scarce resources is not just a necessary, but also a noble, pursuit. After all, in public systems, health care is funded (and therefore owned) by society, and resource allocators who attempt to make the most of resources do so to the benefit of us all. Yet these decision-makers are often pilloried, not just by interest groups, but also by the governments who allocate priority-setting responsibilities to them. In writing this book, we were motivated by a desire to help this group navigate the vagaries of the rationing role and to suggest ways in which this might become a more defensible and less painful process. However, we do not pretend to have the answers, or that these can ever be identified. We hope to have laid out some of the features of effective priority setting, but, ultimately, much will depend on the leadership shown by those taking responsibility for making and implementing tough decisions. In the introduction, we suggested that resource allocation can only take us so far in managing the gap between demand and supply in health care, and that strategies are required for addressing its root causes. To this end, the local priority setter can engage in dialogue designed to bring about more realistic expectations of what can be achieved by public health care systems. However, reducing the rationing gap will require others – government, industry, the clinical community and the public – to play their part. In the meantime, priority setting will remain a necessary but thankless task.

References

Abelson, J., Lomas, J., Eyles, J., Birch, S. and Beenstra, G. (1995) 'Does the community want devolved authority? Results of deliberative polling in Ontario', *Canadian Medical Association Journal*, vol 153, pp 403–12.

Abelson, J., Forest, P., Eyles, J., Smith, P., Martin, E. and Gauvin, F. (2003) 'Deliberations about deliberative methods: issues in the design and evaluation of public participation processes', *Social Science and Medicine*, vol 57, pp 239–51.

Alimo-Metcalfe, B. and Alban-Metcalfe, J. (2005) 'Leadership: time for a new direction?', *Leadership*, vol 1, pp 51–71.

America Speaks (2004) *A Million Voices: a Blueprint for Engaging the American Public in National Policy-Making*, Washington: America Speaks.

Anand, S. (2000) 'The concern for equity in health', *Journal of Epidemiology and Community Health*, vol 56, pp 485–7.

Anand, S. and Hanson, K. (1997) 'Disability-adjusted life years: a critical review', *Journal of Health Economics*, vol 16, pp 685–702.

Appleby, J. (2008) 'The credit crisis and health care', *British Medical Journal*, vol 337, p a2259.

Appleby, J. and Maybin, J. (2008) 'Topping up NHS Care', *British Medical Journal*, vol 337, pp 1122–3.

Appleby J., Crawford R. and Emmerson C. (2009) 'How cold will it be? Prospects for NHS funding 2011–17', London: Kings Fund.

Arnstein, S.R. (1969) 'A ladder of citizen participation', *Journal of the American Institute of Planners*, vol 35, pp 216–24.

Baltussen, R., Stolk, E., Chisholm, D. and Aikins, M. (2006) 'Towards a multi-criteria approach for priority setting: an application to Ghana', *Health Economics*, vol 15, pp 689–96.

Barker, C. (1996) *The Health Care Policy Process*, London: Sage.

Barnes, M., Newman, J. and Sullivan, H. (2007) *Power, Participation and Political Renewal: Case Studies in Public Participation*, Bristol: The Policy Press.

Bate, A. and Mitton, C. (2006) 'Application of economic principles in healthcare priority setting', *Expert Review of Pharmacoeconomics and Outcomes Research*, vol 6, pp 275–84.

Beauchamp, T. and Childress, J. (1989) *Principles of Biomedical Ethics*, Oxford: Oxford University Press.

Belton, V. and Stewart, T.J. (2002) *Multi Criteria Decision Analysis: an Integrated Approach*, The Netherlands: Kluwer.

Bennis, W.G. (1994) *On Becoming a Leader*, New York: Perseus Press.

Berger, P.L. and Luckmann, T. (1966) *The Social Construction of Reality: a Treatise in the Sociology of Knowledge*, Garden City, NY: Anchor Books.

Berney, L., Kelly, M., Doyal, L., Feder, G., Griffiths, C. and Rees Jones, I. (2005) 'Ethical principles and the rationing of health care: a qualitative study in general practice', *British Journal of General Practice*, vol 517, pp 620–5.

Berry, J., Portney, K., Bablitch, M. and Mahoney, R. (1984) 'Public involvement in administration: the structural determinants of effective citizen participation', *Nonprofit and Voluntary Sector Quarterly*, vol 13, pp 7–23.

Birch, S. and Gafni, A. (2006) 'Information created to evade reality (ICER) – things we should not look to for answers', *Pharmacoeconomics*, vol 24, pp 1121–31.

Blaug, K., Horner, L. and Lekhi, R. (2006) *Public Value, Citizen Expectations and User Commitment: a Literature Review*, London: Work Foundation.

Bohmer, P., Pain, C., Watt, A., Abernethy, P. and Sceats, J. (2001) 'Maximising health gain within available resources in the New Zealand public health system', *Health Policy*, vol 55, pp 37–50.

Bolden, R. and Gosling, J. (2006) 'Leadership competencies: time to change the tune?' *Leadership*, vol 2, pp 147–63.

Bots, P.W.G. and Hulshof, A.M. (2000) 'Designing multi-criteria decision analysis processes for priority setting in health policy', *Journal of Multi Criteria Decision Analysis*, vol 9, pp 56–75.

Bowling, A. (1996) 'Health care rationing: the public's debate', *British Medical Journal*, vol 312, pp 670–4.

Brazier, J., Deverill, M., Green, C., Harper, R. and Booth, A. (1999) 'A review of the use of health status measures in economic evaluation', *Health Technology Assessment*, vol 3, pp 1–164.

Briggs, H. (2010) 'Critics condemn bowel cancer drug rejection', *BBC News*, 24 August.

Broome, J. (1991) *Weighing Goods*, Oxford: Basil Blackwell.

Bruni, R., Laupacis, A. and Martin, D. (2008) 'Public engagement in setting priorities in health care', *Canadian Medical Association Journal*, vol 179, pp 15–18.

Buse, K., Mays, N. and Walt, G. (2005) *Making Health Policy*, Maidenhead: Open University Press.

Cabinet Office (2006) *Partnership in Public Services: an Action Plan for Third Sector Involvement*, London: Cabinet Office.

Caiels, J., Forder, J.F., Malley, J., Netton, A. and Windle, K. (2010) *Measuring Outcomes for Public Service Users' Project*, London: PSSRU.

Calabresi, G. and Bobbitt, B. (1979) *Tragic Choices*, New York: Norton.

Callaghan, G. and Wistow, G. (2006) 'Publics, patients, citizens, consumers? Power and decision making in primary health care', *Public Administration*, vol 84, pp 583–601.

Callahan, D. (1988) *Setting Limits: Medical Goals in an Ageing Society*, New York: Touchstone Books.

Caplan, A. (1994) 'Ethics of casting the first stone: personal responsibility, rationing and transplants', *Alcohol: Clinical and Experimental Research*, vol 18, pp 219–21.

Chadwick, R. (1998) 'Management, ethics and the allocation of resource', in S. Dracopoulou (ed) *Ethics and Values in Health Care Management*, London: Routledge.

Chambers, S. (2004) 'Behind closed doors: publicity, secrecy, and the quality of deliberation', *Journal of Political Philosophy*, vol 12, pp 389–410.

Child, J. (1988) *Organization: a Guide to Problems and Practice*, London: Paul Chapman.

Coast, J. (2004) 'Is economic evaluation in touch with society's health values?', *British Medical Journal*, vol 329, pp 1233–6.

Coast, J. and Donovan, J. (1996) 'Conflict, complexity and confusion: the context for priority setting', in J. Coast, J. Donovan and S. Frankel (eds) *Priority Setting: ahe Health Care Debate*, Chichester: Wiley and Sons.

Coast, J., Donovan, J. and Frankel, S. (1996) *Priority Setting: ahe Health Care Debate*, Chichester: John Wiley and Sons.

Cohen, J.P. (2006) 'Cost-effectiveness and resource allocation', *Jama – Journal of the American Medical Association*, vol 295, pp 2723.

Coleman, S. and Gøtze, J. (2002) *Bowling Together: Online Engagement in Policy Deliberation*, London: Hansard Society.

Contandripoulos, D. (2000) 'A sociological perspective on public participation in health care', *Social Science and Medicine*, vol 58, pp 321–30.

Contandripoulos, D., Denis, J.-L., Langley, A. and Valette, A. (2004) 'Governance structures and political processes in a public system: lessons from Quebec', *Public Administration*, vol 82, pp 627–55.

Cooksey, S.D. (2006) *A Review of UK Health Service Research Funding*, London: Her Majesty's Treasury.

Cookson, R. and Dolan, P. (2000) 'Principles of justice in health care rationing', *Journal of Medical Ethics*, vol 26, pp 323–9.

Cookson, R., McCabe, T. and Tsuchiya, A. (2008) 'Public healthcare resource allocation and the rule of rescue', *Journal of Medical Ethics*, vol 34, pp 540–4.

Cooper, C. and Starkey, K. (2010) 'Disinvestment in health care: a shared vocabulary, language, and narrative of change are needed', *British Medical Journal*, no 340, p 605.

Coote, A. and Lenaghan, J. (1997) *Citizen's Juries: Theory into Practice*, London: Institute for Public Policy Research.

Cornforth, C. (2003) *The Governance of Public and Non-Profit Organisations – What Do Boards Do?*, London: Routledge.

Coulter, A. (1999) 'Paternalism or partnership? Patients have grown up and there's no going back', *British Medical Journal*, vol 319, pp 719–20.

Council of Europe (2000) *The Development of Structures for Citizen and Patient Participation in the Decision-Making Process Affecting Health Care. Recommendation 5, Adopted 24/02/2000*, Strasbourg: Council of Europe.

Cunningham, C. (1963) 'Policy and practice', *Public Administration*, vol 41, pp 229–37.

Daniels, N. (1990) *Am I My Parent's Keeper? An Essay on Justice between the Young and Old*, Oxford: Oxford University Press.

Daniels, N. (2000) 'Accountability for reasonableness. Establishing a fair process for priority setting is easier than agreeing on principles', *British Medical Journal*, vol 321, pp 1300–1.

Daniels, N. and Sabin, J. (2008) *Setting Limits Fairly. Learning to Share Resources for Health*, Oxford: Oxford University Press.

Davies, C., Wetherall, M. and Barnett, E. (2006) *Citizens at the Centre: Deliberative Participation in Healthcare Decisions*, Bristol: The Policy Press.

Deakin, N. (1994) *The Politics of Welfare Continuities and Change*, Hemel Hempstead: Harvester Wheatsheaf.

Dennis, A.R., George, L.M., Jessup, J.F., Nunamaker, J.F. and Vogel, D.R. (1988) 'Information technology to support electronic meetings', *MIS Quarterly*, vol 12, pp 591–624.

Department of Health (2009) *World Class Commissioning Handbook*, London: Department of Health.

Department of Health (2010a) 'Programme budgeting categories'. Available at: www.dh.gov.uk/en/Managingyourorganisation/Financeandplanning/Programmebudgeting/index.htm (accessed 3 December 2010).

Department of Health (2010b) *The NHS Constitution*, London: Department of Health.

Dickinson, H. (2008) *Evaluating Outcomes in Health and Social Care*, Bristol: The Policy Press.

Dickinson, H., Glasby, J., Forder, J. and Beesley, L. (2007a) 'Free personal care in Scotland: a narrative review', *British Journal of Social Work*, vol 37, pp 459–74.

Dickinson, H., Glasby, J., Peck, E. and Ham, C. (2007b) 'NHS independence: can things only get better?' *British Journal of Healthcare Management*, vol 13, pp 164–5.

Dickinson, H., Peck, E., Durose, J. and Wade, E. (2010) 'Efficiency, effectiveness and efficacy: towards a framework for high-performance in health care commissioning', *Public Money and Management*, vol 30, pp 167–74.

Dolan, P. (2000) 'The measurement of health-related quality of life for use in resource allocation decisions in healthcare', in A.J. Culyer and J.P. Newhouse (eds) *Handbook of Health Economics, volume 1*.

Dolan, P. and Tsuzhiya, A. (2009) 'The social welfare function and individual responsibility: some theoretical issues and empirical evidence', *Journal of Health Economics*, vol 28, pp 210–20.

Dolan, P., Gudex, C., Kind, P. and Williams, A. (1995) *A Social Tariff for Euroqol: Results from a UK General Population Survey*, York: Centre for Health Economics.

Dolan, P., Cookson, R. and Ferguson, B. (1999) 'Effect of discussion and deliberation on the public's views of priority setting in health care: focus group study', *British Medical Journal*, vol 318, p 919.

Donaldson, C., Bate, A., Mitton, C., Dionne, F. and Ruta, D. (2010) 'Rational disinvestment', *QJM*, vol 103, no 10, pp 801–07..

Douglas, C. and Ammeter, A. (2004) 'An examination of leader political skill and its effect on ratings of leader effectiveness', *The Leadership Quarterly*, vol 15, pp 537–50.

Drummond, M.F., Sculpher, M.J., Torrance, G.W., O'Brien, B.J. and Stoddart, G.L. (2005) *Methods for the economic evaluation of health care programmes* (3rd edn) Oxford: Oxford University Press.

Dryzek, J. (2001) 'Legitimacy and economy in deliberative democracy', *Political Theory*, vol 29, pp 651–69.

Dworkin, R. (2000) *Sovereign Virtue: the Theory and Practice of Equality*, Cambridge, MA: Harvard University Press.

Dye, T. (2001) *Top Down Policymaking*, London: Nelson.

Ecckhoudt, L. (1996) 'Expected utility theory is it normative or simply practical', *Medical Decision Making*, vol 16, pp 12–13.

Eddama, O. and Coast, J. (2009) 'Use of economic evaluation in local health care decision-making in England: a qualitative investigation', *Health Policy*, vol 89, pp 261–70.

Elshaug, A., Hiller, J., Tunis, J. and Moss, J. (2007) 'Challenges in Australian policy processes for disinvestment from existing, ineffective health care practices', *Australia and New Zealand Health Policy*, vol 4, p 23.

Elshaug, A.G., Moss, J.R., Littlejohns, P., Karnon, J., Merlin, T.L. and Hiller, J.E. (2009) 'Identifying existing health care services that do not provide value for money', *Medical Journal of Australia*, vol 190, pp 269–73.

Essink-Bot, M.L., Pereira, J., Packer, C., Schwarzinger, M., Burstrom, K. and European Disability Weights Group (2002) 'Cross-national comparability of burden of disease estimates: the European Disability Weights Project', *Bulletin of the World Health Organization*, vol 80, pp 644–52.

Etzioni, A. (1964) *Modern Organizations*, London: Prentice Hall.

Evans, J. (1997) 'The rationing debate: rationing health care by age: the case against', *British Medical Journal*, vol 314, pp 820–2.

Fairhurst, G.T. (1993) 'Echoes of the vision: how the rest of the organization talks total quality management', *Management Communication Quarterly*, vol 6, pp 331–71.

Fairhurst, G.T. and Chandler, T.A. (1989) 'Social structure in leader member interaction', *Communication Monographs*, vol 56, pp 215–39.

Ferner, R. and McDowell, S. (2006) 'How NICE may be outflanked', *British Medical Journal*, vol 332, pp 1268–71.

Fischhoff, B. (1991) 'Value elicitation – is there anything in there?', *American Psychologist*, vol 46, pp 835–47.

Fishkin, J. (1991) *Democracy and Deliberation*, New Haven: Yale University Press.

Florin, D. and Dixon, J. (2004) 'Public involvement in health care', *British Medical Journal*, vol 328, pp 159–61.

Forster, R. and Gabe, J. (2008) 'Voice or choice? Patient and public involvement in the National Health Service in England under New Labour', *International Journal of Health Services*, vol 38, pp 333–56.

Fox-Rushby, J. (2002) *Disability Adjusted Life Years (Dalys) for Decision Making? An Overview of the Literature*, London: Office of Health Economics.

Friedman, A. (2008) 'Beyond accountability for reasonableness', *Bioethics*, vol 22, pp 101–12.

Gafni, A. and Birch, S. (2006) 'Incremental cost-effectiveness ratios (ICERs): the silence of the lambda', *Social Science and Medicine*, vol 62, pp 2091–100.

Gallego, G., Taylor, SJ., McNeill, P. and Brien, J. (2007) 'Public views on priority setting for High Cost Medications in public hospitals in Australia', *Health Expectations*, vol 10, pp 224–35.

Gallego, G., Haas, M.R., Hall, J.P. and Viney, R.C. (2010) 'Reducing the use of ineffective health care interventions', CHERE Working Paper 2010/5.

Gelijns, A.C., Brown, L.D., Magnell, C., Ronchi, E. and Moskowitz, A.J. (2005) 'Evidence, politics and technological change', *Health Affairs*, vol 24, pp 29–40.

Gemmill, G. and Oakley, J. (1992) 'Leadership: an alienating social myth?', *Human Relations*, vol 45, pp 113–29.

Gibson, J., Martin, D. and Singer, P.A. (2005) 'Priority setting in hospitals: fairness, inclusiveness, and the problem of institutional power differences', *Social Science and Medicine*, vol 61, pp 2355–62.

Gilbert, D. (2007) 'Political challenges for the lay representative', in S. Green (ed) *Involving People in Healthcare Policy and Practice*, Oxford: Radcliffe.

Gillon, R. (1994) 'Medical ethics: four principles plus attention to scope', *British Medical Journal*, vol 309, p 184.

Gilson, L. (2003) 'Trust and the development of health care as a social institution', *Social Science and Medicine*, vol 56, pp 1453–68.

Glasby, J. (ed) (2011) *Commissioning for Health and Well-Being: an Introduction*, Bristol: The Policy Press.

Glasby, J. and Dickinson, H. (2008) *Partnership Working in Health and Social Care*, Bristol: The Policy Press.

Glasby, J., Walshe, K. and Harvey, G. (2007a) *Evidence Based Practice*, Special edition of *Evidence and Policy*, vol 3, no 3, pp 323-457.

Glasby, J., Peck, E., Ham, C. and Dickinson, H. (2007b) *'Things Can Only Get Better?' The Argument for NHS Independence*, Birmingham: Health Services Management Centre.

Goddard, M., Hauck, K., Preker, A. and Smith, P. (2006) 'Priority setting in health – a political economy perspective', *Health Economics, Policy and Law*, vol 1, pp 79–90.

Gold, M.R. (2005) 'Tea, biscuits, and health care prioritizing', *Health Affairs*, vol 24, pp 234–9.

Gold, M.R., Siegel, J.E., Russell, L.B. and Weinstein, M.C. (1996) *Cost-Effectiveness in Health and Medicine*, New York: Oxford University Press.

Goodin, R. and Pettit, P. (2006) *Contemporary Political Philosophy: an Anthology*, Oxford: Blackwell.

Grant, W. (1984) 'The role of pressure groups', in R. Borthwick and J. Spence (eds) *British Politics in Perspective*, Leicester: Leicester University Press.

Grint, K. (2000) *The Arts of Leadership*, Oxford: Oxford University Press.

Grint, K. (2005a) 'Problems, problems, problems: the social construction of "leadership"', *Human Relations*, vol 58, pp 1467–94.

Grint, K. (2005b) *Leadership: Limits and Possibilities*, Basingstoke: Palgrave Macmillan.

Guston, D. (1999) 'Evaluating the first US consensus conference: the impact of the citizens' panel on telecommunications and the future of democracy', *Science, Technology and Human Values*, vol 24, pp 451–82.

Gutmann, A. and Thompson, D. (2004) *Why Deliberative Democracy?*, New Jersey: Princeton University.

Gwatkin, D. (2000) 'Health inequalities and the health of the poor: what do we know?', *Bulletin of the World Health Organization*, vol 78, pp 3–17.

Hadorn, D. (1991a) 'Setting health care priorities in Oregon: Cost-effectiveness meets the rule of rescue', *Journal of American Medical Association*, vol 265, pp 2218–25.

Hadorn, D.C. (1991b) 'The Oregon priority-setting exercise – quality-of-life and public-policy', *Hastings Center Report*, vol 21, pp S11–S16.

Ham, C. and Coulter, A. (2000) 'International experiences of rationing (or priority setting)', in A. Coulter and C. Ham (eds) *The Global Challenge of Health Care Rationing*, Buckingham: Open University Press.

Ham, C. and Coulter, A. (2001) 'Explicit and implicit rationing: taking responsibility and avoiding blame for health care choices', *Health Services Research and Policy*, vol 6, pp 163–9.

Ham, C. and Dickinson, H. (2008) *Engaging Doctors in Leadership: What Can We Learn from International Experience and Research Evidence?*, Warwick: NHS Institute for Innovation and Improvement.

Ham, C. and Pickard, S. (1998) *Tragic Choices in Health Care: the Case of Child B*, London: Kings Fund.

Ham, C. and Robert, G. (2003) *Reasonable Rationing: International Experiences of Priority Setting in Health Care*, Maidenhead: Open University Press.

Harding, M. (2005) 'Hewitt, Herceptin and the £100 million bill PCTs can't afford to pay', *Health Service Journal*, December.

Harris, J. (1987) 'QALYfying the value of life', *Journal of Medical Ethics*, vol 13, pp 117–23.

Harrison, S. (1998) 'The politics of evidence-based medicine in the United Kingdom', *Policy and Politics*, vol 26, pp 15–31.

Harrison, S. and Mort, M. (1998) 'Which champions, which people? Public and user involvement in health care as a technology of legitimation', *Social Policy and Administration*, vol 32, pp 60–70.

Hartley, J. and Bennington, J. (2010) *Leadership for Healthcare*, Bristol: The Policy Press.

Hartley, J. and Branicki, L. (2006) *Managing with Political Awareness: a Summary Review of the Literature*, London: Chartered Management Institute.

Hartley, J., Fletcher, C., Wilton, P., Woodman, P. and Ungemach, C. (2007) *Leading with Political Awareness: Developing Leaders' Skills to Manage the Political Dimension across Sectors*, London: Chartered Management Institute.

Hasman, A. and Holm, S. (2005) 'Accountability for reasonableness: opening the black box of process', *Health Care Analysis*, vol 13, pp 261–73.

Hauck, K., Smith, P.C. and Goddard, M. (2003) *The Economics of Priority Setting for Health Care: a Literature Review*, Washington: World Bank.

Heath, I. (1999) '"Uncertain clarity": contradiction, meaning and hope', *British Journal of General Practice*, vol 49, pp 651–7.

Heginbotham, C. (1993) 'Health care priority setting: a survey of doctors, managers and the general public', in *Rationing in Action*, London: BMJ publishing.

Henderson, J., Roberts, T.E., Sikorski, J., Wilson, J. and Clement, S. (2000) 'An economic evaluation comparing two schedules of antenatal visits', *Journal of Health Services Research and Policy* 5, 69–75.

Hewison, A. (2004) 'Evidence-based management in the NHS: is it possible?', *Journal of Health Organisation and Management*, vol 18, pp 336–48.

Hinscliff, G. (2008) 'Hospitals deny IVF treatment to smokers', *The Observer*, 22 June.

Hirschberg, S., Dones, R. and Heck, T. (2004) *Sustainability of Electricity Supply Technologies under German Conditions: a Comparative Evaluation*, Switzerland: Paul Scherrer Institut.

Hogg, C. (2007) 'Patient and public involvement: what next for the NHS?', *Health Expectations*, vol 10, pp 129–38.

Holm, S. (1998) 'Goodbye to the simple solutions: the second phase of priority setting in health care', *British Medical Journal*, vol 317, pp 1000–2.

Hope, T. (2001) 'Rationing and life-saving treatments: should identifiable patients have higher priority?', *Journal of Medical Ethics*, vol 27, pp 179–85.

Huff, A. (1988) 'Politics and argument as a means of coping with ambiguity and change', in L.R. Pondy, R.J. Boland and H. Thomas (eds) *Managing Ambiguity and Change*, New York: John Wiley.

Humphries, R., Forder, J.F. and Fernandez, J. (2010) *Securing Good Care for More People: Options for Reform*, London: Kings Fund.

Hunter, D. (1997) *Desperately seeking solutions*, Longman: London.

Ibargoyen-Roteta, N., Gutierrez-Ibarlueza, I., Asua, J., Benguria-Arrate, G. and Galnares-Cordero, L. (2009) 'Scanning the horizon of obsolete technologies: possible sources for their identification', *International Journal of Technology Assessment in Health Care*, vol 25, pp 249–54.

Independent Commission (2004) *The Good Governance Standards for Public Services*, London: Office for Public Management and Chartered Institute of Public Finance and Accountancy.

Iredale, R. and Longley, M. (1999) 'Public involvement in policy-making: the case of a Citizens' Jury on genetic testing for common disorders', *Journal of Consumer Studies and Home Economics*, vol 23, pp 3–10.

Jagsi, R., DeLaney, T., Donelan, K. and Tarbell, N. (2004) 'Real-time rationing of scarce resources: the Northeast Proton Therapy Centre experience', *Journal of Clinical Oncology*, vol 22, pp 2246–50.

Jenkings, K.N. and Barber, N. (2004) 'What constitutes evidence in hospital new drug decision making?', *Social Science and Medicine*, vol 58, pp 1757–66.

Jessop, B. (2003) 'Governance and metagovernance: on reflexivity, requisite variety, and requisite irony', in H. Bang (ed) *Governance, as Social and Political Communication*, Manchester: Manchester University Press.

Jones, I. (2004) 'Is patient involvement possible when decisions involve scarce resources? A qualitative study of decision-making in primary care', *Social Science and Medicine*, vol 59, pp 93–102.

Jones, K. (2008) 'In whose interest? Relationships between health consumer groups and the pharmaceutical industry in the UK', *Sociology of Health and Illness*, vol 30, pp 929–43.

Jonsen, A. (1986) 'Bentham in a box: technology assessment and health care allocation', *Law, Medicine and Health Care*, vol 14, pp 172–4.

Joss, S. and Durant, J. (1995) *Consensus Conferences in Europe*, London: Science Museum.

Kahneman, D. and Smith, V. (2002) *Foundations of Behavioural and Experimental Economics*, Stockholm: The Royal Swedish Academy of Sciences.

Kapiriri, L., Norheim, O. and Martin, D. (2009) 'Fairness and accountability for reasonableness. Do the views of priority setting decision makers differ across health systems', *Social Science and Medicine*, vol 68, pp 766–73.

Kershaw, B. (2006) 'Performance studies and Po-Chang's ox: steps to a paradoxology of performance', *NTQ*, vol 22, pp 30–53.

Klein, R. (1984) 'The politics of participation', in R. Maxwell and N. Weaver (eds) *Public Participation in Health*, London: King Edward's Hospital Fund.

Klein, R. (2010) 'Rationing in the fiscal ice age', *Health Economics, Policy and Law*, vol 5, pp 389–96.

Klein, R. and Williams, A. (2000) 'Setting priorities: what is holding us back – inadequate information or inadequate institutions?', in A. Coulter and C. Ham (eds) *The Global Challenge of Health Care Rationing*, Buckingham: Open University Press.

Klein, R., Day, P. and Redmayne, S. (1996) *Managing Scarcity: Priority Setting and Rationing in the National Health Service*, Maidenhead: Open University Press.

Kmietowicz, Z. (2006) 'NICE is to root out ineffective treatments in NHS', *British Medical Journal*, vol 333, p 568.

Knapp, M. (1999) 'Economic evaluation and mental health: sparse past … fertile future?', *Journal of Mental Health Policy and Economics*, vol 2, pp 163–7.

Knights, D. and O'Leary, M. (2005) 'Reflecting on corporate scandals: the failure of ethical leadership', *Business Ethics: A European Review*, vol 14, pp 359–66.

Kondro, W. and Sibbald, B. (2005) 'Patient demand and politics push Herceptin forward', *Canadian Medical Association Journal*, vol 1723, pp 347–8.

Kovner, A.R., Elton, J.J. and Billings, J.D. (2000) 'Evidence-based management', *Frontiers of Health Services Management*, vol 16, pp 3–24.

Kruijshar, M., Barendregt, J. and the European Disability Weights Group (2004) 'The breast cancer related burden of morbidity and mortality in six European countries: the European Disability Weights project', *European Journal of Public Health*, vol 14, pp 141–6.

Light, D. (1997) 'The real ethics of rationing', *British Medical Journal*, vol 315, pp 112–15.

Litva, A., Coast, J., Donovan, J., Eyles, J., Shepherd, M., Tacchi, J., Abelson, J. and Morgan, L. (2002) 'The public is too subjective: public involvement at different levels of health-care decision making', *Social Science and Medicine*, vol 54, pp 1825–37.

Locock, L. (2000) 'The changing nature of rationing in the UK National Health Service', *Public Administration*, vol 78, pp 91–109.

Lomas, J. (1997) 'Reluctant rationers: public input into health care priorities', *Journal of Health Services Research and Policy*, vol 2, pp 103–11.

Lomas, J., Culyer, T., McCutcheon, C., McAuley, L. and Law, S. (2005) *Conceptualizing Evidence for Health System Guidance: Final Report*, Ottawa: Canadian Health Research Foundation.

Lootsma, F.A. (1999) 'The expected future of MCDA', *Journal of Multi Criteria Decision Analysis*, vol 8, pp 59–60.

Loughlin, M. (1998) 'Impossible problems? The limits to the very idea of reasoning about the management of health services', in S. Dracopoulou (ed) *Ethics and Values in Health Care Management*, London: Routledge.

Luskin, R., Fishkin, J. and Jowell, R. (2002) 'Considered opinion: deliberative polling in Britain', *British Journal of Policy*, vol 32, pp 455–87.

Lynn, L., Heinrich, C. and Hill, C. (2001) *Improving Governance: a New Logic for Empirical Research*, Washington DC: Georgetown University Press.

Mabey, C. and Finch-Lees, T. (2008) *Management and Leadership Development*, London: Sage Publications Ltd.

MacKenzie, R., Chapman, S. and Salkeld, G. (2008) 'Media influence on Herceptin subsidization in Australia: application of the rule of rescue?', *Journal of the Royal Society of Medicine*, vol 101, pp 305–12.

Mansbridge, J. (2010) 'Deliberative polling as the gold standard', *The Good Society*, vol 19, pp 55–62.

Marmot Commission (2010) *Fair Society, Healthy Lives: The Marmot Review*, London: The Marmot Review.

Martin, G.P. (2008) 'Representativeness, legitimacy and power in public involvement in health-care management', *Social Science and Medicine*, vol 67, pp 1757–65.

Matland, R.E. (1995) 'Synthesizing the implementation literature: the ambiguity–conflict model of policy implementation', *Journal of Public Administration Research and Theory*, vol 5, pp 145–74.

Maynard, A. (2001) 'Ethics and health care "underfunding"', *Journal of Medical Ethics*, vol 27, pp 223–7.

Mays, N. (2000) 'Legitimate decision making: the Achilles' heel of solidaristic health care systems', *Journal of Health Services Research and Policy*, vol 5, pp 122–6.

McCabe, C., Claxton, K. and Tsuchiya, A. (2005) 'Orphan drugs and the NHS: should we value rarity?', *British Medical Journal*, vol 331, p 1016.

McDaid, D., Byford, S. and Sefton, T. (2003) *Because It's Worth It: a Practical Guide to Conducting Economic Evaluations in the Social Welfare Field*, York: Joseph Rowntree Foundation.

McGuire, A. (2001) 'Theoretical concepts in the economic evaluation of health care', in M.F. Drummond and A. McGuire (eds) *Economic Evaluation in Health Care*, Oxford: Oxford University Press.

McIver, S. (1998) *Health Debate? An Independent Evaluation of Citizens Juries in Health Settings*, London: Kings Fund.

McKenzie, J. (2001) *Perform or Else: From discipline to performance*, London: Routledge.

McKie, J. and Richardson, J. (2003) 'The rule of rescue', *Social Science and Medicine*, vol 56, pp 2407–19.

Mechanic, D. (1995) 'Dilemmas in rationing health care services: the case for implicit rationing', *British Medical Journal*, vol 310, pp 1655–9.

Mendoza, G.A. and Martins, H. (2006) 'Multi-criteria decision analysis in natural resource management: a critical review of methods and new modelling paradigms', *Forest Ecology and Management*, vol 230, pp 1–22.

Menon, D., Stafinski, T. and Martin, D. (2007) 'Priority-setting for healthcare: who, how and is it fair?', *Health Policy*, vol 84, pp 220–33.

Michailakis, D. and Schirmer, W. (2010) 'Agents of their health? How the Swedish welfare state introduces expectations of individual responsibility', *Sociology of Health and Illness*, vol 32, pp 930–47.

Milewa, T. and Barry, C. (2005) 'Health policy and the politics of evidence', *Social Policy and Administration*, vol 39, pp 498–512.

Milewa, T., Valentine, J. and Calnan, M. (1999) 'Community participation and citizenship in British health care planning: narratives of power and involvement in the changing welfare state', *Sociology of Health and Illness*, vol 21, pp 445–65.

Mitton, C. and Donaldson, C. (2001) 'Twenty-five years of programme budgeting and marginal analysis in the health sector 1974–1999', *Journal of Health Services Research and Policy*, vol 6, pp 239–48.

Mitton, C. and Donaldson, C. (2003) 'Resource allocation in health care: health economics and beyond', *Health Care Analysis*, vol 11, pp 245–57.

Mitton, C., Donaldson, C. and Manderville, P. (2003) 'Priority setting in a Canadian long-term care setting: a case study using program budgeting and marginal analysis', *Canadian Journal on Aging – Revue Canadienne du Vieillissement*, vol 22, pp 311–21.

Mitton, C., Smith, N., Peacock, S., McEvoy, B. and Abelson, J. (2009) 'Public participation in health care priority setting: a scoping review', *Health Policy*, vol 91, pp 219–28.

Mooney, G. (1998) '"Communitarian claims" as an ethical basis for allocating health care resources', *Social Science and Medicine*, vol 4, pp 1171–80.

Moore, A. (2010) 'PCTs restrict many treatments as overspend looms', *Health Service Journal* December 2, p 12.

Morgan, M. (2005) *Classics of Moral and Political Theory*, Indianapolis: Hackett Publishing.

Muir Gray, J.A. (1997) *Evidence-Based Health Care: How to Make Health Policy and Management Decisions*, New York: Churchill Livingstone.

Mullen, P. (1999) 'Public involvement in health care priority setting: an overview of methods for eliciting values', *Health Expectations*, vol 2, pp 222–34.

Mullen, P. and Spurgeon, P. (2000) *Priority Setting and the Public*, Oxon: Radcliffe Medical Press.

Murray, C.J., Salomon, J.A. and Mathers, C. (2000) 'A critical examination of summary measures of population health', *Bulletin of the World Health Organization*, vol 78, pp 981–94.

Netten, A., Forder, J., Beadle-Brown, J., Caiels, J., Malley, J., Smith, N., Towers, A., Trukeschitz, B., Welch, E. and Windle, K. (2010) *ASCOT Adult Social Care Outcomes Tool Kit*, Kent: PSSRU.

Newdick, C. and Derrett, S. (2006) 'Access, equity and the role of rights in health care', *Health Care Analysis*, vol 14, pp 157–68.

NHS Oxfordshire (2010) 'Priorities forum'.

NICE (National Institute for Health and Clinical Excellence) (2006) *Citizens Council Report: Rule of Rescue*, London: NICE.

NICE (2007) *Bevacizumab and Cetuximab for the Treatment of Metastatic Colorectal Cancer*, London: NICE.

NICE (2008) *Social Value Judgements: Principles for the Development of NICE Guidance*, London: NICE.

NICE (2010) *Measuring Effectiveness and Cost Effectiveness: The QALY*, London: NICE.

Niessen, l.W., Grijseels, E.W.M. and Rutten, F.F.H. (2000) 'The evidence based approach in health policy and health care delivery', *Social Science and Medicine*, vol 51, pp 859–69.

Nord, E. (1991) 'The validity of a visual analogue scale in determining social utility weights for health states', *International Journal of Planning and Management*, vol 6, pp 234–42.

Nord, E. (2005) 'Concerns for the worse off: fair innings versus severity', *Social Science and Medicine*, vol 60, pp 257–63.

Norheim, O.F. (1999) 'Healthcare rationing – are additional criteria needed for assessing evidence based clinical practice guidelines?', *British Medical Journal*, vol 319, pp 1426–9.

Nunamaker, J.F., Briggs, R.O., Mittleman, D.D. and Vogel, D.R. (1997) 'Lessons from a dozen years of group support systems research: a discussion of lab and field findings', *Journal of Management Information Systems*, vol 13, pp 163–207.

Nuti, S., Vainieri, M. and Bonini, A. (2010) 'Disinvestment for re-allocation: a process to identify priorities in healthcare', *Health Policy*, vol 95, pp 137–43.

Olsen, J. (1997) 'Theories of justice and their implications for priority setting in health care', *Journal of Health Economics*, vol 16, pp 625–39.

Organisation for Economic Co-operation and Development (2004) 'OECD principles of corporate governance'. Available at: www.oecd.org/topic/0,337 3,en_2649_37439_1_1_1_1_37439,00.html (accessed 8 October 2010).

Osborne, S.P. and Kinder, T. (2011) '"Want doesn't get"? Public management responses to the recession', *Public Money and Management*, vol 31, pp 85–8.

Øvretveit, J. (1995) *Purchasing for Health: a Multi-Disciplinary Introduction to the Theory and Practice of Purchasing*, Buckingham: OUP.

Øvretveit, J. (1997) 'Managing the gap between demand and publicly affordable health care in an ethical way', *European Journal of Public Health*, vol 7, p 128.

Palmer, S. and Torgerson, D.J. (1999) 'Economics notes – definitions of efficiency', *British Medical Journal*, vol 318, p 1136.

Parkinson, J. (2004) 'Why deliberate? The encounter between deliberation and new public managers', *Public Administration*, vol 2, pp 377–95.

Parry, G., Moysera, G. and Day, N. (1992) *Political Participation and Democracy in Britain*, Cambridge: Cambridge University Press.

Paul, C., Nicholls, R., Priest, P. and McGee, R. (2008) 'Making policy decisions about population screening for breast cancer: the role of citizens' deliberation', *Health Policy*, vol 85, pp 314–20.

Payne, J.W., Bettman, J.R. and Johnson, E.J. (1992) 'Behavioral decision research: a constructive processing perspective', *Annual Review Psychology*, vol 43, pp 87–131.

Peacock, S., Mitton, C., Bate, A., McCoy, B. and Donaldson, C. (2009) 'Overcoming barriers to priority setting using interdisciplinary methods', *Health Policy*, vol 92, nos 2-3, pp 124–32.

Peck, E. and Dickinson, H. (2008) *Managing and Leading in Inter-Agency Settings*, Bristol: The Policy Press.

Peck, E. and Dickinson, H. (2009) *Performing Leadership*, Basingstoke: Palgrave Macmillan.

Peterson, M. (1999) 'Motivation, mobilisation and monitoring: the role of interest groups in health policy', *Journal of Health Politics, Policy and Law*, vol 24, pp 416–20.

Phillips, L.D. (2007) 'Decision conferencing', in W. Edwards, R. Miles and D. von Winterfeldt (eds) *Advances in Decision Analysis: from Foundations to Applications*, New York: Cambridge University Press.

Piccart-Gebhart, M., Procter, M. and Leyland-Jones, B. (2005) 'Trastuzumab after adjunct chemotherapy in HER2-positive breast cancer', *New England Journal of Medicine*, vol 353, pp 1659–72.

Pidd, H. (2010) 'Avastin prolongs life but drug is too expensive for NHS patients, says NICE', *The Guardian*. Available at: www.guardian.co.uk (accessed 12 October 2010).

PSSRU (Personal Social Services Research Unit) (2010) *Adult Social Care Outcomes Tool-kit (ASCOT)*, www.pssru.ac.uk/ascot

Rawlins, M. and Culver, A. (2004) 'National Institute for Clinical Excellence and its value judgements', *British Medical Journal*, vol 329, pp 224–7.

Rawls, J. (1971) *A Theory of Justice*, Oxford: Oxford University Press.

Reeleder, D., Goel, V., Singer, P.A. and Martin, D.K. (2006) 'Leadership and priority setting: the perspective of hospital CEOs', *Health Policy*, vol 79, pp 24–34.

Rein, M. and Schön, D.A. (1993) 'Reframing policy discourse', in F. Fischer and J. Forester (eds) *The Argumentative Turn in Policy Analysis and Planning*, Durham, NC: Duke University Press.

Richardson, J. (2002) 'The poverty of ethical analysis in economics and the unwarranted disregard of evidence', in C. Murray and A. Lopez (eds) *Summary Measures of Population Health*, Geneva: World Health Organisation.

Right Care (2010) 'The NHS atlas of variation in healthcare'. Available at: www.rightcare.nhs.uk

Roberts, T.E., Robinson, S., Barton, P.M., Bryan, S., McCarthy, A., Macleod, J., Egger, M. and Low, N. (2007) 'Cost-effectiveness of home based population screening for Chlamydia trachomatis in the UK: economic evaluation of chlamydia screening studies (ClaSS)', *British Medical Journal*, vol 355.

Robinson, R. (1999) 'Limits to rationality: economics, economists and priority setting', *Health Policy*, vol 49, pp 13–26.

Robinson, S. (2011) 'Financing healthcare: funding systems and healthcare costs', in K. Walshe and J. Smith (eds) *Health Care Management*, Basingstoke: Open University Press/McGraw Hill.

Robinson, S., Dickinson, H. and Williams, I. (2009) *Evaluation of the Prioritisation Process at South Staffordshire PCT*, Birmingham: Health Services Management Centre.

Robinson, S., Dickinson, H., Freeman, T. and Williams, I. (2011a) 'Disinvestment in health: the challenges facing general practitioner (GP) commissioners', *Public Money and Management*, vol 31, pp 145–8.

Robinson, S., Dickinson, H., Williams, I., Freeman, T., Rumbold, B. and Spence, K. (2011b) *Setting Priorities in Health: a Study of English Primary Care Trusts*, London: The Nuffield Trust

Romond, E., Perez, E. and Bryant, J. (2005) 'Trastuzumab plus adjunct chemotherapy for operable HER-2 positive breast cancer', *New England Journal of Medicine*, vol 353, pp 1673–84.

Rowe, G. and Frewer, L. (2005) 'A typology of public engagement mechanisms', *Science, Technology and Human Values*, vol 30, pp 251–90.

Rowe, R. and Shepherd, M. (2002) 'Public participation in the new NHS: no closer to citizen control?', *Social Policy and Administration*, vol 36, pp 275–90.

Russell, G. and Greenhalgh, R. (2009) *Rhetoric, Evidence and Policymaking: a Case Study of Priority Setting in Primary Care. Final Report of a Research Project Funded by the UCL Leverhulme–ESRC Programme on Evidence, Inference and Enquiry*, London: University College London.

Ruta, D., Mitton, C., Bate, A. and Donaldson, C. (2005) 'Programme budgeting and marginal analysis: bridging the divide between doctors and managers', *British Medical Journal*, vol 330, pp 1501–3.

Ryynanen, O., Myllykangas, M., Kinnunaqn, J. and Takala, J. (1999) 'Attitudes to health care prioritisation methods and criteria among nurses, doctors, politicians and the general public', *Social Science and Medicine*, vol 49, pp 1529–39.

Sabik, L. and Lie, R. (2008) 'Priority setting in health care: lessons from the experiences of eight countries', *International Journal for Equity and Health*, vol 7 (published online).

Sabin, J. (1998) 'Fairness as a problem of love and the heart: a clinician's perspective on priority setting', *British Medical Journal*, vol 317, pp 1002–4.

Sackett, D.L., Richardson, W.S., Rosenberg, W. and Haynes, R. (1997) *Evidence-Based Medicine: How to Practice and Teach EBM*, Edinburgh: Churchill Livingstone.

Samuelson, P.A. (1980) *Economics: an Introductory Analysis*, New York: McGraw-Hill Company.

Schedler, P. and Glastra, F. (2001) 'Communicating policy in late modern society: on the boundaries of interactive policy making', *Policy and Politics*, vol 29, pp 337–49.

Schlander, M. (2008) 'The use of cost-effectiveness by the National Institute for Health and Clinical Excellence (NICE): no(t yet an) exemplar of a deliberative process', *Journal of Medical Ethics*, vol 34, pp 534–9.

Schöne-Seifert, B. (2009) 'The "rule of rescue" in medical priority setting: ethical plausibilities and implausibilities', *Rationality, Markets and Morals*, vol 0, pp 421–30.

Schwappach, D. and Koeck, C. (2004) 'Preferences for disclosure: the case of bedside rationing', *Social Science and Medicine*, vol 59, pp 1891–7.

Schwartzman, H. (1989) *The Meeting: Gatherings in Organisations and Communities*, New York: Plenum.

Secretary of State for Health (2000) *The NHS Plan: the Government's Response to the Royal Commission on Long Term Care*, London: The Stationery Office.

Secretary of State for Health (2010) *Equity and Excellence: Liberating the NHS*, London: HSMO.

Shapiro, J. (2010) 'The NHS: the story so far (1948–2010)', *Clinical Medicine, Journal of the Royal College of Physicians*, vol 10, pp 336–8.

Shiell, A., Hawe, P. and Seymour, J. (2000) 'Will our understanding of completeness ever be complete?', *Health Economics*, vol 9, pp 729–31.

Shotter, J. (1999) *Conversational Realities*, London: Sage Publications.

Sibbald, S.L., Singer, P.A., Upshur, R. and Martin, D.K. (2009) 'Priority setting: what constitutes success? A conceptual framework for successful priority setting', *Bmc Health Services Research*, vol 9.

Simon, H.A. (1978) 'Rationality as process and as product of thought', *American Economic Review*, vol 68, pp 1–16.

Simon, H. (1997 [1945]) *Administrative Behaviour: a Study of Decision-Making Processes in Administrative Organisations*, New York: Free Press.

Singer, P. and Mapa, J. (1998) 'Ethics of resource allocation: dimensions for healthcare executives', *Hospital Quarterly*, vol 1, pp 29–31.

Singer, P., Martin, D., Giacomini, M. and Purdy, L. (2000) 'Priority setting for new technologies in medicine: qualitative case study', *British Medical Journal*, vol 321, pp 1316–18.

Skelcher, C., Mathur, N. and Smith, M. (2004) *Effective Partnership and Good Governance: Lessons for Policy and Practice*, University of Birmingham: Institute of Local Government Studies.

Smircich, L. and Morgan, G. (1982) 'Leadership and the management of meaning', *Journal of Applied Behavioral Science*, vol 18, pp 257–73.

Smith, G. and Wales, C. (2000) 'Citizens juries and democracy', *Political Studies*, vol 48, pp 51–65.

Smith, J., Curry, N., Mays, N. and Dixon, J. (2010) *Where Next for Commissioning in the English NHS?*, London: The Nuffield Trust.

South Central Priorities Support Unit (2008) 'South Central ethical framework', available from www.oxfordshirepct.nhs.uk

Southwark PCT (2009) *Policy on prioritisation for investment and disinvestment in health services, Board papers*, Southwark: Southwark Primary Care Trust.

Stewart, T.J. (1992) 'A critical survey of the status of multiple criteria decision making theory and practice', *Omega*, vol 20, pp 569–86.

Sulmasy, D. (1992) 'Physicians, cost control, and ethics', *Annals of Internal Medicine*, vol 116, pp 920–6.

Syrett, K. (2003) 'A technocratic fix to the "legitimacy problem"? The Blair government and health care rationing in the United Kingdom', *Journal of Health Politics, Policy and Law*, vol 28, pp 715–46.

Tannenbaum, S. (1994) 'Knowing and acting in medical practice: outcomes research', *Journal of Health Politics, Policy and Law*, vol 19, pp 27–44.

Tauber, A. (2002) 'Medicine, public health and the ethics of rationing', *Perspectives in Biology and Medicine*, vol 45, pp 16–30.

Tenbensel, T. (2002) 'Interpreting public input into priority setting: the role of mediating institutions', *Health Policy*, vol 62, pp 173–94.

The Committee on the Financial Aspect of Corporate Governance and Gee and Co Ltd (1992) *The Financial Aspects of Corporate Governance*, London: Gee.

The Health Foundation (2010) *Improvement in Practice: Commissioning with the Community*, London: Health Foundation.

The Lancet (2005) 'Herceptin and early breast cancer: a moment for caution', *The Lancet*, vol 366, pp 1673.

The Sun (2009) 'No NHS drug for tumour dad, 37', *The Sun*, 20 October.

Thompson, A. (2007) 'The meaning of patient involvement and participation in health care consultations: a taxonomy', *Social Science and Medicine*, vol 64, pp 1297–310.

Times Online (2008) 'Change your lifestyle if you want to have treatment on the NHS', *Times Online*, 1 October. Available at: www.thetimes.co.uk (accessed 23 November 2010).

Torrance, G. (1971) 'A generalised cost-effectiveness model for the evaluation of health programs', doctoral dissertation, State University of New York at Buffalo.

Torrance, G.W. (1986) 'Measurement of health state utilities for economic appraisal', *Journal of Health Economics*, vol 5, pp 1–30.

Tritter, J. and McCallum, A. (2006) 'The snakes and ladders of user involvement: moving beyond Arnstein', *Health Policy*, vol 76, pp 156–68.

Tsuchiya, A. and Dolan, P. (2005) 'The QALY model and individual preferences: a systematic review of the literature', *Medical Decision Making*, vol 25, no 54, pp 460–7.

Twaddle, S. and Walker, A. (1995) 'Program budgeting and marginal analysis – application within programs to assist purchasing in Greater Glasgow Health Board', *Health Policy*, vol 33, pp 91–105.

Ubel, P., Arnold, R. and Caplan, A. (1993) 'Rationing failure: the ethical lessons of the retransplantation of scarce vital organs', *Journal of American Medical Association*, vol 270, pp 2469–74.

van Stokkom, B. (2005) 'Deliberative group dynamics: power status and affect in interactive policy making', *Policy and Politics*, vol 33, pp 387–409.

Vergel, Y. and Ferguson, B. (2006) 'Difficult commissioning choices: lessons from English primary care trusts', *Journal of Health Services Research and Policy*, vol 11, pp 150–4.

von Neumann, J. and Morgenstern, O. (1944) *Theory of Games and Economic Behaviour*, Princeton: Princeton University Press.

Wagstaff, A. (1991) 'QALYs and the equity–efficiency trade-off', *Journal of Health Economics*, vol 10, pp 21–41.

Waite, S. and Nolte, E. (2006) 'Public involvement policies in health: exploring their conceptual basis', *Health Economics, Policy and Law*, vol 1, pp 149–62.

Wall, A. (1998) 'Ethics and management – oil and water?', in S. Dracopoulou (ed) *Ethics and Values in Health Care Management*, London: Routledge.

Wanless, D. (2004) *Securing Good Health for the Whole Population: Final Report*, London: HM Treasury, Crown.

Wanless, D. (2006) *Securing Good Care for Older People: Taking a Long Term View*, London: Kings Fund.

Weale, A. (1995) 'The ethics of rationing', *British Medical Bulletin*, vol 51, pp 831–41.

Weick, K.E. (1995) *Sensemaking in Organisations*, Thousand Oaks, CA: Sage.

Weinstein, M.C. and Stason, W. (1977) 'Foundations of cost-effectiveness analysis for health and medical practices', *New England Journal of Medicine*, vol 296, pp 716–21.

Weiss, C. (1979) 'The many meanings of research utilization', *Public Administration Review*, vol 39, pp 426–31.

Williams, A. (1985) 'Economics of coronary artery bypass grafting', *British Medical Journal*, vol 291, pp 326–9.

Williams, A. (1992) 'Cost-effectiveness analysis: is it ethical?', *Journal of Medical Ethics*, vol 18, pp 7–11.

Williams, A. (1997) 'Intergenerational equity: an exploration of the fair innings argument', *Health Economics*, vol 6, pp 117–32.

Williams, A. (1998) 'Economics, QALYs and medical ethics: a health economist's perspective', in S. Dracopoulou (ed) *Ethics and Values in Health Care Management*, London: Routledge.

Williams, A. (1999) 'Calculating the global burden of disease: time for a strategic reappraisal', *Health Economics*, vol 8, pp 1–8.

Williams, I. (2009) *Cost-Effectiveness Analysis and Technology Coverage Decision Making. The Case of the English NHS*, Birmingham: University of Birmingham.

Williams, I. (2011) 'Allocating resources for healthcare: setting and managing priorities', in K. Walshe and J. Smith (eds) *Healthcare Management*, Maidenhead: Open University Press.

Williams, I. and Bryan, S. (2007a) 'Cost-effectiveness analysis and formulary decision making in England: findings from research', *Social Science and Medicine*, vol 65, pp 2116–29.

Williams, I. and Bryan, S. (2007b) 'Understanding the limited impact of economic evaluation in health care resource allocation: a conceptual framework', *Health Policy*, vol 80, pp 135–43.

Williams, I. and Dickinson, H. (2010) 'Can knowledge management enhance technology adoption in health care? A review of the literature', *Evidence and Policy*, vol 6, pp 309–31.

Williams, I., Dickinson, H. and Robinson, S. (2011a) 'Joined-up rationing? The role of priority setting in health and social care commissioning', *Journal of Integrated Care*, vol 10, issue 1, pp 3–11.

Williams, I., Phillips, D., Nicholson, C. and Shearer, H. (2011b) 'Citizen deliberation and priority setting in the English NHS', unpublished.

Wiseman, V., Mooney, G., Berry, G. and Tang, K. (2003) 'Involving the general public in priority setting: experiences from Australia', *Social Science and Medicine*, vol 56, pp 1001–12.

World Health Organization (2000) *The World Health Report 2000. Health Systems: Improving Performance*, Geneva: World Health Organization.

Yang, K. (2005) 'Public administrators' trust in citizens: a missing link in citizen involvement efforts', *Public Administration Review*, May/June, pp 3–273.

Yeo, M., Williams, J. and Hooper, W. (1999) 'Incorporating ethics in priority setting: a case study of a rational health board in Canada', *Health Care Analysis*, vol 7, pp 177–94.

Young, I.M. (2000) *Inclusion and Democracy*, Oxford: Oxford University Press.

Index